Diabetic Lifestyle:

Diabetic Medical Food Book and Diabetic Diet.

Best Way to Reverse Diabetes with Diabetic Plate Recipes.

by

Viktoria McCartney

Legal & Disclaimer

The information contained in this book and its contents is not designed to replace or take the place of any form of medical or professional advice; and is not meant to replace the need for independent medical, financial, legal, or other professional advice or services, as may be required. The content and information in this book have been provided for educational and entertainment purposes only.

The content and information contained in this book have been compiled from sources deemed reliable, and it is accurate to the best of the Author's knowledge, information, and belief. However, the Author cannot guarantee its accuracy and validity and cannot be held liable for any errors and/or omissions. Further, changes are periodically made to this book as and when needed. Where appropriate and/or necessary, you must consult a professional (including but not limited to your doctor, attorney, financial advisor or such other professional advisor) before using any of the suggested remedies, techniques, or information in this book.

Upon using the contents and information contained in this book, you agree to hold harmless the Author from and against any damages, costs, and expenses, including any

Table of Contents

Introduction

Diabetes, known as diabetes mellitus, is a metabolic disorder. A metabolic disorder is one that affects the normal chemical processes in the body and results in an imbalance in some of the core body and cellular functions on the molecular level. In the case of diabetes mellitus, it is the control and regulation of blood glucose levels within the optimum range that is impaired. There is a normal psychological range which our body maintains the blood glucose levels in. Beyond that range, as in an increase or decrease outside the normal physiological value, results in an imbalance in the concentration of blood glucose that causes the metabolic disorder known as diabetes. This eventually results in an imbalance in several metabolic pathways in several organs and the deposition of excess glucose in organs where it is not supposed to be deposited.

Diabetes is an imbalance in the amount of glucose in the blood as a result of a defect in the regulation of the metabolism of glucose, and its consequent removal from the blood and storage in an insoluble form. There are lots of tedious details about our body's regulatory system and how it regulates our blood glucose level and strives to keep it constant within the physiological range. However, these details are beyond the scope of this book. What is important to discuss in this book is how our habits, especially our eating habits can result in a shift in our blood glucose levels outside the normal range and how by including certain food and avoiding certain foods we can control, to an extent, our blood glucose level and try to maintain it within the normal level. When the body's regulatory system fails, it becomes our responsibility to keep the level of our glucose in our blood in check, we must take conscious steps to take charge of the situation. Before we discuss the habits you can modify, let us understand more about the biology of diabetes, how to identify it, and how to live with it.

The Biological Background of Diabetes

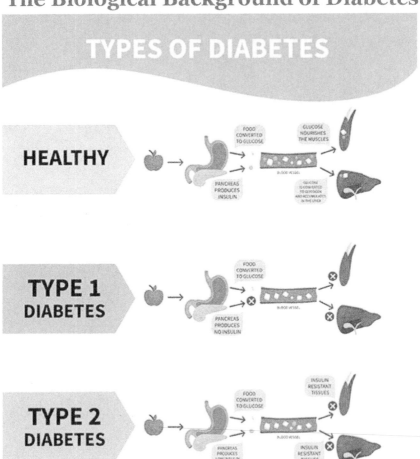

TYPES OF DIABETES

The Journey of Glucose

When you eat food, especially food that contains carbohydrates or starch, you ingest polysaccharides which get digested and broken down into sugars, specifically glucose. The digested glucose gets absorbed by your small intestines and into the blood. From there it travels around the body to supply the different cells in the various organs of your body.

Why Sugar is Important

All cells need glucose in order to survive. The glucose is the main food of the cells as it is the fuel that cells burn in respiration to release energy which every cell needs to maintain its life processes. Without adequate nutrition, especially glucose, cells will malfunction and eventually die if the glucose starvation prolongs.

On the contrary, if the blood contains lots of excessive glucose for long periods of time on a consistent basis, your blood starts to dump the excess sugars into healthy cells and tissues in abundance where the sugar is not supposed to be deposited. This deposition of sugar into tissues where it's not supposed to be affects the function of the different organs and results in all the complications of diabetes, which can be annoying to live with. As you can see it works both ways any deviation from the normal physiological blood glucose levels results in undesirable effects that affect the health of your organs and consequently your health overall.

The Need for Controlling Blood Glucose Levels

It is important to control blood glucose levels because when the amount of glucose in the blood exceeds the normal range for prolonged periods of time it results in problems in several organs of our body. These are the complications of uncontrolled diabetes which we will discuss shortly. Similarly, when the blood glucose levels drops below the normal, your body doesn't get its adequate supply of energy and therefore it is also not healthy to have lower than normal blood glucose levels. We will now discuss the biological background of diabetes.

For that reason, the body has developed a mechanism to monitor and control the blood glucose levels. Normally this involves cells that constantly measure the amount of blood glucose. These are cells in the pancreas, and they can measure the blood glucose as the blood passes through the pancreas during its circulation. When the cells in the pancreas detect an abnormal level of glucose, whether above or below the normal, it wants to communicate this important finding with other responsible organs that will take control of the situation.

They communicate via chemical messengers called hormones. When hormones are released, they travel through the blood and go to their target organ and signal specific information that tells the organ it is time to do a certain task. It is already pre-programmed in each cell what each hormone is designed to inform that target cell.

Normally the pancreas upon detecting an abnormal amount of blood glucose, releases either insulin or glucagon hormones depending on whether the level was above or below the normal. The target organ for these hormones is the liver which upon receiving the signal works to either increase or decrease the blood glucose level to bring it back to normal.

When the blood glucose level is above normal, the special pancreatic cells release the hormone insulin which travels in the blood to reach its target organ, the liver, and instructs it to absorb some glucose from the blood. The liver then transforms the excess glucose, which is in the soluble form, into an insoluble form known as glycogen.

The liver then stores this excess glycogen. Since glycogen is insoluble, it does not affect the osmotic balance in the media where it is stored. The media where glycogen is stored refers to the fluid inside the cells that contains many stored products, including insoluble glycogen and even glucose. The problem with excess glucose is that it is soluble. That means it affects the concentration of the liquid in which it is in, whether in the blood or in the cells. The blood and the fluid inside the cells need to be in a specific concentration for the cell to have an optimum environment to perform all its physiological functions. When there is excess glucose in the blood or in the cells, it affects the concentration of the fluid.

Think about a glass of water with just one spoon of sugar and another glass with 5 spoons of sugar. Eventually, the excess sugar ruins the consistency of the fluid and lumps up as it is unable to dissolve completely. This is what happens in the blood and cells when they have excess glucose that they are not able to get rid of (when their regulatory mechanisms fail, as in diabetes).

Therefore, in excess blood sugar states, the insulin signals the liver to remove the soluble glucose and transform it into an insoluble form which will not cause a shift in the concentration of the fluid it is in.

Glucagon is the hormone released by the pancreatic cells which monitor the blood glucose levels when it detects that the blood glucose level is below the normal range. This hormone instructs the liver to break down some of its stored glycogen back into glucose and release it to the blood which was low on glucose.

When the pancreas is healthy, it can detect blood glucose level and produce insulin any time the blood glucose level rises to maintain the glucose levels within the normal physiological range.

If, for example, you eat a meal that is full of sweets and carbohydrates your level of glucose in the blood is going to rise significantly. This results in an increase in the secretion of insulin to further speed up the conversion of glucose into glycogen and eventually restore the normal blood glucose as soon as possible. Put differently, a healthy pancreas can adapt its production of insulin to match the increased amount of blood glucose at any given time.

Diabetes is a long-term imbalance in the regulation of blood glucose level. There is often a fault in one or more parts in the mechanism of blood glucose regulation. This fault can be genetic or acquired. It can be that the cells that detect the blood glucose levels cannot detect the levels accurately, or in other words, they have become insensitive to the difference in blood glucose levels. Or they can detect the difference, but they are unable to produce insulin or enough insulin.

As mentioned above a healthy pancreas can match the release of insulin with the degree of the rise of glucose. A certain type of diabetes might be able to produce insulin but may not be able to produce just enough to meet increased demands, for example, after a highly sugary meal.

What are Some of the Factors that Affect our Blood Glucose Levels

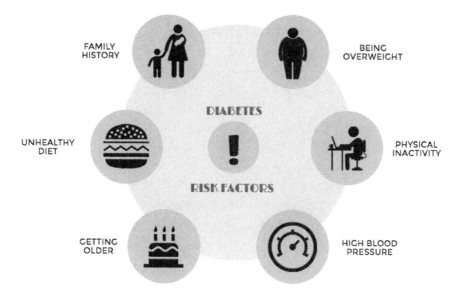

There are several factors that can affect your blood glucose levels. Being fully aware of these allows you to have better control and management of your diabetes.

Your Level of Physical Activity

Physical activity and exercise have a significant effect on your blood glucose levels. For example, physical exercise can affect insulin sensitivity for up to 2 days from the exercise, leading to a reduction in blood glucose levels over this time. On the short term, bursts of activity will result in a rise in sugar levels as the body is trying to compensate for the increased demand for glucose by releasing more glucose into the blood.

Studies have shown that if you exercise on the muscle that is close to where you have injected your insulin, this could lead your insulin to be absorbed quickly, therefore, affecting your glucose levels.

The number of carbs and proteins you ingest also affects your sugar level as proteins eventually get broken down into glucose. Carbs obviously get broken down into glucose more frequently and regularly than proteins.

Your Alcohol Intake

Your alcohol intake also affects your blood glucose levels. Alcohol intake greatly increases the risk of developing hypoglycemia which is low blood sugar levels. Avoid drinking alcohol on an empty stomach as this will quickly and rapidly increase the amount of alcohol in your blood. Avoid binge drinking or continuous drinking as all this can increase the risk of developing hypoglycemia which can be threatening.

Where you Inject your Insulin

The location where you inject your insulin also effects how fast it is absorbed. It would help if you were careful to regularly change up your injection sites to ensure that the insulin is distributed and absorbed consistently all over your body. Lumpy skin can affect the absorption of the injection. Therefore, it is important to rotate your injection sites to avoid developing lumpy skin. It is advised to inject into regions of your body that have a decent layer of fat. Examples include the belly, your thighs, buttocks and upper arms. The quickest area where insulin gets absorbed from is the belly then the upper arm and then the thighs and lastly in the buttocks. If you have skinny arms injecting into your arm might not be the best injection option as you may end up injecting your insulin into a muscle and this can lead to hyperglycemia.

Studies have shown that it is for the best to inject in the same general area when it comes to the same type of meal. For example, if you inject in your stomach for breakfast, inject each day in your stomach for breakfast. For lunch, you can inject in your upper arm and keep it that way for all lunches.

Other Factors

Other factors that could affect your blood glucose levels are the menstrual cycle of women, pregnancy, and other medications that may be treating other diseases that interfere with the blood glucose levels. If you suffer from gastroparesis which is characterized by delayed emptying of the stomach this can have an impact; as well as things like missing out a dose of your insulin or glucose regulating medication. All these factors can impact upon your glucose levels which is why you need to take into account the varying factors that will affect your blood glucose levels.

Understanding Diabetes Type 2

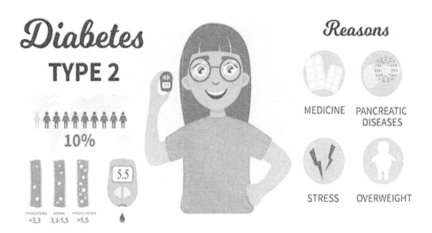

Type 2 diabetes is the commonest type of diabetes with about 90% of diabetics being type 2. This is an acquired form of diabetes. That is why it usually develops later in life in adults although the recent trend has shown in younger people and even sometimes children developing this disease. This is in contrast with type 1 diabetes which is genetic and therefore manifests early in life.

This type 2 of diabetes occurs when your body is resisting the effects of insulin and becomes unresponsive to the signaling of the hormone. That is, when insulin is signaling the liver as well as other cells to absorb some of the excess glucose and the cells are unable to receive or appropriately interpret the signal of insulin. This is known as insulin resistance.

It can also be due to the inability to produce enough insulin to match the increased levels of glucose due to acquired pancreatic exhaustion or infection that led to permanent damage. Either way, both conditions lead to higher than normal blood glucose levels.

SYMPTOMS OF TYPE 2 DIABETES

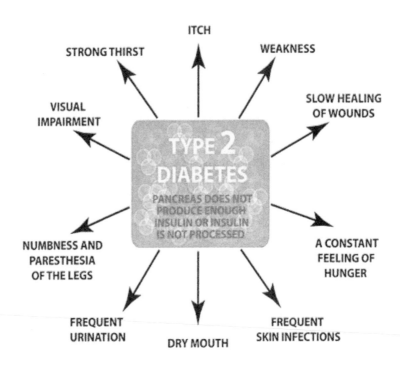

Excessive Thirst

Water is essential for many of our bodily functions. That is why feeling thirsty is a protective mechanism to help us drink an adequate amount of water. However, excessive thirst could be a symptom of developing diabetes. It is worth noting that there are many conditions that cause fluid loss that will cause physiological excessive thirst. For example, eating salty or spicy food, having profuse sweating, vomiting and diarrhea or certain medications.

All this can induce excessive thirst. Therefore, not every excessive thirst is an indication of high blood glucose levels or developing diabetes. Nevertheless, excessive thirst is one of the big signs of diabetes mellitus. Excessive thirst is defined as having persistent and unexplained thirst despite how much water you drink, while also passing more than 5 liters of urine per day.

Frequent Urination

Frequent urination, also known as polyuria, is defined as passing large amounts of urine, usually more than 3 liters per day. The average adult urine output per day is 1 to 2 liters. One of the main symptoms of developing diabetes is having frequent urination.

Frequent urination is caused due to the excessive drinking of water that occurs with diabetes. Moreover, this happens because when the kidney filters blood, normally all the glucose would be returned to the bloodstream. However, in diabetes, some of the blood glucose passes down with the urine and therefore, this draws out more water. This results in an abnormally large volume of urine.

It is important to note that there are other causes for polyuria including kidney disease, liver failure, pregnancy and other medical conditions. If you are frequently urinating, you can test out your sugar levels using glucose testing strips. You will test positive for glucose in urine if you have diabetes.

However, you must confirm this diagnosis with your GP and blood tests done at the pathology lab.

Increased Appetite

Polyphagia or increased appetite is a term used when you are feeling excessive hunger and is one of the main symptoms of diabetes. Excessive hunger can be explained if you have been doing strenuous exercise or have been dealing with stress or depression. Although polyphagia is one of the main three symptoms along with increased thirst and frequent urination that causes you to suspect diabetes, polyphagia can also be caused by other conditions such as premenstrual syndrome, binge eating disorder, bulimia, stress, anxiety and being on corticosteroid medications, etc.

The excessive hunger can be explained by the cells' insulin resistance which means that the cells cannot absorb the glucose from the blood so they cannot use it as a fuel to release the energy they need. This lack of energy results in an increased hunger as the cells are signaling the body to ingest more food in order to provide them with the energy they need. However, the problem is not in the lack of food, but it is in fact in the inability of cells to use the glucose that is circulating in the blood.

In this case, it is counterproductive to eat more as it will not control the situation. In fact, it will increase the already high blood glucose levels. It is advised to decrease the blood glucose levels by exercising and this can stimulate the cells in the pancreas to produce insulin in diabetes type 2 and reduce the blood sugar levels further.

The key symptom to differentiate polyphagia from having extreme hunger is that it does not go away by eating more food or eating more than the normal. If you notice a sudden increase in appetite, perhaps it is time to consult your doctor.

Constant Fatigue

Fatigue is the term used to describe extreme exhaustion and tiredness that doesn't go away with sleeping or resting. There are obviously many reasons for feeling fatigue, on top of them is lack of sleep as we need between 6 to 8 hours of continuous sleep in order to feel well rested. Other conditions that cause fatigue include anemia, depression, cancer and celiac disease and of course, diabetes.

Insulin resistance is caused by the high blood sugar levels resulting in the cells having energy deficits and being unable to meet the energy requirements. This leads you to feel tired and lacking energy overall. To identify fatigue, it is defined as the lack of energy which manifests in having difficulty in carrying out simple everyday tasks. Moreover, you can also have mental fatigue by feeling down and depressed.

You can try regular exercise along with a healthy diet and a good night's sleep to boost your energy levels. For mental fatigue, you can try mindfulness and other meditation-based techniques to overcome stress and depression and elevate your mental health. If you are having extreme fatigue that is not due to lack of sleep and that has persisted for 3 to 4 weeks, it is important to visit your doctor and seek medical advice.

Weight Loss or Losing Muscle Mass

Having sudden and unexplained weight loss is often an alarming sign. Your ideal weight is determined by several factors, including your calorie intake, age, level of physical activity and your overall health. During childhood and puberty, your weight can change rapidly. However, during adulthood years, your weight remains relatively stable year by year. Unexplained weight loss that did not occur due to dieting or exercise should be investigated medically.

Weight loss occurs due to the high levels of glucose and the insulin resistance. Which causes the body cells to be unable to gain the energy they need from glucose. As a result, they start burning fats or muscles to release the energy they need. This results in a reduction in your body mass by losing fat and muscle mass.

Slow Wound Healing

The accumulation of excess sugars affects the nerves and results in poor blood circulation. This affects skin repair which is manifested by poor wound healing. Wounds can remain unhealed and open for prolonged periods of time, leading to fungal and bacterial infections and further complications.

Blurred Vision

Blurred vision is one of the symptoms of diabetes that is when you lose the sharpness of your vision and the inability to see the fine details. You can have blurred vision in one eye or both eyes. There are of course several other reasons that can cause blurred vision. However, diabetes is one of the differential diagnosis causing blurred vision. The high levels of sugar cause the lens inside your eyes to swell, and when it does, it affects the quality of your eyesight. Blurred vision is defined as the inability to see fine details or form a sharp image.

Management of Diabetes Type 2

TYPE 2 DIABETES
MANAGEMENT

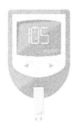

blood glucose level
monitoring

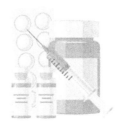

diabetes medication
or insulin therapy

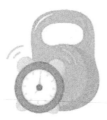

regular physical activity

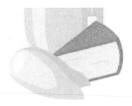

healthy diet

The first line of treatment for people who have diabetes type 2 is a combination of modification of dietary habits and regular, moderate exercise. The medical guidelines recommend having a diet that is low on the glycemic index, high in fiber and low in carbohydrates. People with type 2 diabetes may have to resort to prescribed tablets or injectable medications in addition to lifestyle modifications. Metformin is one of the key drugs for treating diabetes type 2 and it encourages the body to respond better to insulin. The doctor will inform you about your medication options if you need it or if you can simply manage your case with only lifestyle modifications.

Examples of the Available Medications

Alpha-glucosidase inhibitors. These are responsible for slowing down carb digestion.

Amylin analogues. These helps the insulin to control blood glucose levels after meals.

Biguanides. These stops the production of glucose in the liver.

Dpp-4 inhibitors. These stops incretin hormones from being broken down.

Incretin mimetics. These help to copy the action of the body's incretin hormone.

Prandial glucose regulators. These helps the pancreatic cells to produce insulin.

SGLT2 inhibitors. These work on the kidneys to decrease blood glucose.

Thiazolidinediones. These help to reduce the body's resistance to insulin.

This is not an exhaustive list of all diabetes' medications. Your GP is the best one fit to decide which medication you should take and the doses according to your case.

Understanding Diabetes Type 1

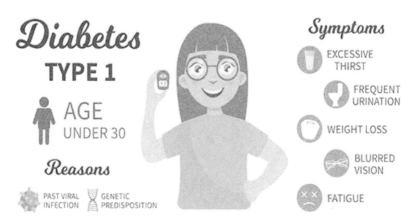

Diabetes type 1 is a genetic, autoimmune condition that starts at an early age. The real trigger is not known for sure, however, a combination of genetic and environmental triggers have been attributed to causing the immune system to start the course of diabetes type 1. In diabetes type 1, the immune system attacks the cells in the pancreas that are responsible for producing insulin. Over time, all the cells in the pancreas that produce insulin die off and the pancreas becomes unable to produce insulin ever again.

When to Suspect Diabetes Type 1

SYMPTOMS OF TYPE 1 DIABETES

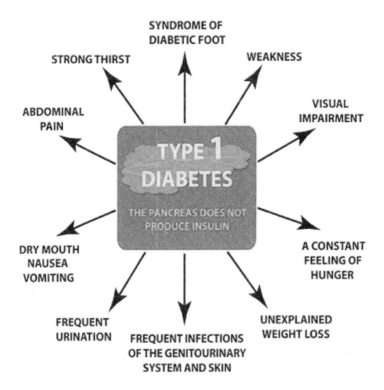

The warning symptoms of diabetes type 1 are the same as type 2, however, in type 1, these signs and symptoms tend to occur slowly over a period of months or years, making it harder to spot and recognize. Some of these symptoms can even occur after the disease has progressed.

Management of Type 1 Diabetes

TYPE 1 DIABETES
MANAGEMENT

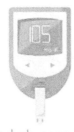

blood glucose level monitoring

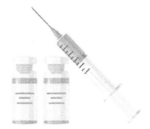

lifelong insulin injections

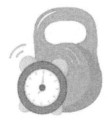

regular physical activity

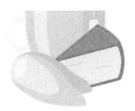

healthy diet

Unfortunately, being diagnosed with type 1 diabetes means that it is essential to be treated with insulin. Insulin injections are found in multiple forms, including rapid acting, long acting, etc. In addition to insulin, it is important to control diabetes by taking conscious care of your dietary habits as well as staying physically active. Sadly, unlike diabetes type 2, lifestyle modifications alone are not enough to substitute the need for insulin injections.

The Different Types of Insulin

Rapid-acting insulin. (Known as Lispro). It reaches the blood quickly, within 15 minutes post injection. Its levels peak from 30 to 90 minutes after that and can last in the blood for as long as 5 hours.

Short-acting (the regular) insulin. This usually reaches the blood shortly within 30 minutes post injection. Its levels peak in the blood from 2 to 4 hours and remains in the blood for approximately 4 to 8 hours.

Intermediate acting (Known as NPH and Lente) insulins injections take 2 to 6 hours to appear in the blood after injection. They take 4 to 14 hours to peak but remain in the blood for about 14 to 20 hours.

Long acting (ultralente) insulin injection needs from 6 to 14 hours to bei functioning. It doesn't have a peak or shows a very small peak during 10 to 16 hours post the injection. However, it remains in the blood from 20 to 24 hours which makes it a suitable option for some cases.

You should discuss with your doctor which form is the best for you and your preferences.

Who is at Risk of Developing Diabetes?

Each disorder has risk factors that when found in an individual, favor the development of the disease. Diabetes is no different. Here are some of the risk factors for developing diabetes.

Having a Family History of Diabetes

Usually having a family member, especially first-degree relatives could be an indicator that you are at risk to develop diabetes. Your risk of developing diabetes is about 15% if you have one parent with diabetes while it is 75% if both your parents have diabetes.

Having Prediabetes

Being pre-diabetic means that you have higher than normal blood glucose levels. However, they are not high enough to be diagnosed as type 2 diabetes. Having pre-diabetes is a risk factor for developing type 2 diabetes as well as other conditions such as cardiac conditions. Since there are no symptoms or signs for prediabetes, it is often a latent condition that is discovered accidentally during routine investigations of blood glucose levels or when investigating other conditions.

Being Obese or Overweight

Your metabolism, fat stores and eating habits when you are overweight or above the healthy weight range contributes to abnormal metabolism pathways that put you at risk for developing diabetes type 2. There have been consistent research results of the obvious link between developing diabetes and being obese.

Having a Sedentary Lifestyle

Having a lifestyle where you are mostly physically inactive predisposes you to a lot of conditions including diabetes type 2. That is because being physically inactive causes you to develop obesity or become overweight. Moreover, you don't burn any excess sugars that you ingest which can lead you to become prediabetic and eventually diabetic.

Having Gestational Diabetes

Developing gestational diabetes which is diabetes that occurred due to pregnancy (and often disappears after pregnancy) is a risk factor for developing diabetes at some point.

Ethnicity

Belonging tocertain ethnic groups such as Middle Eastern, South Asian or Indian background. Studies of statistics have revealed that the prevalence of diabetes type 2 in these ethnic groups is high. If you come from any of these ethnicities, this puts you at risk of developing diabetes type 2 yourself.

Having Hypertension

Studies have shown an association between having hypertension and having an increased risk of developing diabetes. If you have hypertension, you should not leave it uncontrolled.

Extremes of Age

Diabetes can occur at any age. However, being too young or too old means your body is not in its best form and therefore, this increases the risk of developing diabetes.

That sounds scary. However, diabetes only occurs with the presence of a combination of these risk factors. Most of the risk factors can be minimized by taking action. For example, developing a more active lifestyle, taking care of your habits and attempting to lower your blood glucose sugar by restricting your sugar intake. If you start to notice you are prediabetic or getting overweight, etc., there is always something you can do to modify the situation. Recent studies show that developing healthy eating habits and following diets that are low in carbs, losing excess weight and leading an active lifestyle can help to protect you from developing diabetes, especially diabetes type 2, by minimizing the risk factors of developing the disorder.

Preventing the Complications of Diabetes

Diabetes, being a metabolic syndrome, has some nasty complications which we will discuss shortly. There are several things that you can do in order to delay or prevent the occurrences of these complications.

Control your HbA1C within Normal Range

HbA1C refers to hemoglobin that has been glycated. This happens when hemoglobin that is a protein inside the red blood cells that is responsible for carrying oxygen throughout your body binds with glucose and therefore becomes glycated.

It would make sense that the more glucose that is available in the blood for long periods of time, the more tendency it has to bind with the circulating hemoglobin in the blood. That is why HbA1C is a measure for doctors to get an overall picture about how your average blood glucose levels have been over the period of few weeks up to a couple of months.

HbA1C is an important and great indicator of the relative risk of developing diabetes related complications. The higher the value of HbA1C, the higher the risk of developing some serious diabetes related complications.

This measure is an accurate average measurement as the glucose in the bloodstream is naturally attracted to the glucose in the blood. Therefore, the amount of glycated hemoglobin will be directly proportional to the total amount of sugar that was inside your blood around that time.

Since the average survival rate of the human red blood cells is 8-12 weeks before they get destroyed and renewed, the measurement of HbA1C is useful in reflecting your average blood glucose levels over that duration, therefore indicating how well you have been controlling and managing your blood glucose in the long-term. In simple words, if your blood glucose levels were high for the past few weeks, your HbA1C will also be high.

Diabetics usually have a 6.5 percentage of HbA1C percentage. This percentage reflects the general recommendation for the diabetic population. However, each person's recommendations should be based on several personal parameters.

Normal HbA1C is approximately 42 mmol/mol

For pre diabetics, it is about 6.2-6.4% or 42 to 47 mmol/mol

For diabetes, it is almost 6.5 or 48 mmol/mol or over

Studies have shown that improving your HbA1C by just 1% for diabetics reduces the risk of having microvascular complications by 25%. Microvascular complications include complications related to retinopathy, nephropathy and neuropathy.

Reducing your hba1c level in people with diabetes type 2 has beenshown to result in a 90% reduction in the risk of developing cataracts, a 16% reduction in the risk of developing heart failure and a 43% risk reduction of suffering from amputation due to peripheral vascular disease.

The key difference between measuring HbA1C and the normal blood glucose instead, is that it measures longer trend whereas the single glucose test reflects a single point in time, that is the time the test was taken.

Losing Weight

Another way you can prevent the complications of diabetes is to lose weight. According to studies, type 2 diabetes is closely linked with being overweight. In fact, over 90% of the recently diagnosed diabetes type 2 patients have been categorized as overweight.

Being overweight not only has physical effects on your body but it also takes a toll on your mental health and your self-esteem therefore losing weight could help you both on the physical level and on the emotional level, especially if you have been already diagnosed with diabetes. It is important that you take some steps to lose weight.

The first step is to know how much you deviate from your ideal weight by measuring yourself and checking the charts. Identify what the healthy weight for your height and age is. Once confronted with the fact, it is important to set the intention to lose weight and remain motivated. You can seek professional guidance or subscribe to a gym or seek a special trainer to help you with your weight loss journey. It is very important to be aware of how obesity and being overweight really affect the progression of your diabetes and how your condition could be much better if you fall back to the normal ideal weight for your age and height group

Control Your Dietary Habits

One of the most important things you can do to control and manage your diabetes to prevent its complications is to take care of your dietary habits. It is impossible to manage your diabetes without controlling and having an appropriate diet. If you have been recently diagnosed with diabetes, it is important to seek advice from a dietitian who will inform you about the different types of diets and which one is suitable for you. There are tons of diets, for example, the Atkins diet, a low carb diet, the 5:2 diet, a low carb high fat diet, meal replacement diet plans, a vegetarian diet, the Dukan diet, a gluten-free diet, a detox diet, the acid alkaline diet, the South Beach diet, a vegan diet, a very low calorie diet, the ketogenic diet and the zone diet.

Become Physically Active

Another thing you can do to decrease your risk of developing complications is to become physically active with exercise. The degree, type and amount of physical activity that you should do while having diabetes should be discussed with your doctor or with advice from a physician. Physical activity has multifold benefits on your health as a person with diabetes. You can lose weight, therefore reducing the risk of disease progression associated with obesity. It also helps to keep your body in burning state, therefore, decreasing your blood glucose levels. In addition, exercise also increases insulin sensitivity for a couple of hours post exercise. There is no specific activity that is best to practice as it varies from one person to another. However, aerobic exercises, training for flexibility and strength, all combined make a very well-rounded exercise routine.

Examples of aerobic exercises are ones that will make your heart beat fast as well as increase your breathing rate. It improves air circulation and gets oxygen as well as glucose to your muscles and therefore, reduces the glucose levels in the blood. Exercising for about 30 minutes per day, five times a week will make a significant difference in your health. Examples of aerobic exercise include dancing, aerobic dance moves, even ice skating and tennis.

Strength training can be very effective for diabetics as building muscles means that more calories get burned as muscles burn more calories than regular tissues. This can be effective in managing diabetes as large amounts of sugars get burned on average.

Stretching and being physically fit and flexible would also help you to prevent joint injuries and leave you feeling mentally superior.

Don't underestimate how much being physically active can improve your overall health, prevent the progression of complications and successfully manage your diabetes. Take a leap of faith and get physically active.

Quit Smoking

One of the important things you can do if you are diabetic to prevent complications is to quit smoking. Not only is smoking associated with a wide range of health conditions such as strokes, several cancers, heart disease as well as increasing the risk of developing the complication of diabetes. It is not an easy task to quit smoking; however, it is not an impossible one. Many ex-smokers have successfully quitted through willpower alone. However, if you are unable to successfully quit relying on willpower alone, there are other smoking cessation aids that can help you — for example, hypnosis, acupuncture, and going to group quitting therapy.

Complications of Diabetes

There are many complications of diabetes. It is worth mentioning some of the key complications that have serious effects as well as persist in high prevalence.

Cardiovascular Complications

One of the key complications of having diabetes is the development of heart disease if diabetes was not well managed for long periods of time. Unfortunately, about 80% of diabetics die from coronary heart disease, but fortunately, the heart attacks that are experienced can be avoided by simple modifications in the lifestyle and taking conscious control of the diabetes condition.

It is a common misconception that cardiovascular diseases only affects the middle-aged and elderly. However, critical cardiovascular disorders can affect diabetics before they reach the age of 30. Both diabetics type 1 and type 2 are at great risk of developing cardiac diseases.

The excess blood glucose levels, in addition to the presence of free fatty acids in the blood causes a change in the walls of blood vessels and leads to the deposition of atherosclerosis and debris which eventually lead to cardiovascular disease. These changes lead to thickening of the vessel wall and obstruction of the blood flow, potentiating heart problems as well as strokes.

Warning symptoms of developing heart disease include stabbing pain in the chest, pain radiating to the left arm, feeling shortness of breath, feeling irregular or rapid heartbeats that do not subside and having swollenfeet or ankles. In order to make sure your heart health is optimum, it is important to take some screening tests, including an ECG, also known as an electrocardiogram.

Two variations of coronary heart disease can manifest, Angina and heart attacks, which are also known as myocardial infarction.

Angina is one of the symptoms of developing coronary heart disease and can be in the form of stable or unstable angina.

People who suffer from stable angina may start to feel discomfort or pain in the chest, that is composed of tightness, dullness or heavy pain that goes away in a couple of minutes. This pain may be associated with triggers such as stress, cold weather, physical or emotional triggers.

On the contrary, unstable angina lasts for more than 5 minutes and persist even if there were no triggers available. If you start to experience angina symptoms, dial your local ambulance service.

The other variant is myocardial infarction or heart attack which is usually caused by a clot that formed either in the heart itself or somewhere else and migrated to the heart and obstructed the blood supply to the heart. The symptoms are usually sharp stabbing pain and strong tightness in the chest associated with shortness of breath coughing and deep feeling of anxiety. If you suspect that you or someone else is having a heart attack, call the emergency services (ambulance) for immediate medical help.

If you have been diagnosed with coronary heart disease, you will be recommended to make some lifestyle modifications.

For example, smoking cessation, improving your lipid profile, eating a healthy and balanced diet, and becoming more physically active each day. You may also be given medications to control your situation such as statins, low dose aspirin, calcium channel blockers or ACE inhibitors.

Diabetic Retinopathy

Diabetic retinopathy is damage to the retina of the eye as a complication of diabetes; it happens when the high blood sugar levels affect the health of your retina. Diabetic retinopathy is also aggravated and develops faster when there is concurrent hypertension. Managing your blood glucose levels and consistently checking your HbA1C is necessary for preventing diabetic retinopathy as the excess blood glucose can damage the blood vessels of the retina which leads to abnormal bleeding in the retina or other issues with the retinal blood vessels.

Diabetic retinopathy screening tests

You can do this once per year at the ophthalmology clinic to spot and recognize early signs of diabetic retinopathy. The goal is not to allow it to develop as, if diabetic retinopathy develops, it can lead to blindness; therefore, it is very critical to schedule an annual retinal exam for screening onceper year.

If you have been diagnosed with diabetes and you are over 12 years old, you should receive an annual retinal exam as per the guidelines. In this exam, the optician will give you eye drops that will dilate your pupils. These eye drops may take up to 20 minutes to dilate your pupils before you are ready for an exam. During the exam, the doctor will take a photo of your retina to view its condition. It is a very painless procedure; however, due to the dilation of your pupils, you may need to avoid driving or crossing the roads as it can be quite difficult due to the expanded pupils. Your pupils will return to their normal size shortly.

If you start to suspect having diabetic retinopathy, you need to go for a screening checkup. Some of the symptoms include distorted or blurred vision, seeing floaters in your vision or sudden changes in your vision or reduction in night vision or even loss of vision.

Cataracts

Although diabetic retinopathy is the most common presentation related to eye-based diabetes complication, there are other conditions that can occur such as glaucoma or cataracts. The unfortunate news is that people who have diabetes have double the risk ofsuffering from glaucoma or cataracts than the general population.

Cataracts are the development of cloudy opacities around the lens of your eyes. This leads to distorted and blurred vision. You can suspect cataracts when you start to have spots on your vision, being dazzled by bright light, seeing yellowing in your vision or having a cloudy or Misty vision. Cataracts can be treated easily by widely acceptable measures due to advancements in medicine.

Glaucoma

Glaucomais another problem that can occur as a result of diabetes, this happens when excess fluid presses on the nerve that is responsible for your vision, called the optic nerve.

Normally, there are chambers in the eye that allow the fluid inside your eyes to drain into a network and leave the eyes, into the bloodstream, so that the eye is gently moist but not overflowing with fluid.

The drainage network system could be clogged due to excess sugar, and the fluid can become trapped inside the eyes. This causes fluid pressure to build up in the eye and press on the nerve at the back of the eye. As a result, the nerve may become damaged by glaucoma. A simple eye exam to measure the pressure in the eye and checking it at the level of the optic nerve and testing field of vision can easily detect glaucoma.

The good news is that the tight control of your diabetes can reduce the risk of development of diabetic eye problems including diabetic retinopathy cataracts or glaucoma.

Another common complication among people with diabetes is the affection of the kidney in a condition that is known as diabetic nephropathy. According to statistics, about 40% of the population of people with diabetes develop nephropathy; however, it is possible to delay or even stop the development of nephropathy via the tight control of blood glucose levels and blood pressure.

The diabetic nephropathy refers to the worsening of the physiological function of kidneys as a result of diabetes; this is often at an advanced level (the fifth and final stage) called end-stage renal disease.. However, it takes about 20 years for diabetic patients to become stage 5 nephropathy. Diabetic nephropathy affects both type 1 and type 2 diabetic patients.

If you see some of the following symptoms you may start to suspect renal affection. These symptoms start to emerge around stage 4 of the diabetic nephropathy disease progression.

You will start a notice that your urine is darker, caused by blood in the urine. You may also start to notice swelling of the ankles and your lower leg or even your hands that is due to edema caused by the retention of water. Your kidney is also responsible for releasing a hormone called erythropoietin. Erythropoietin is responsible for the proper development of red blood cells which carry oxygen in your blood to all your living cells and tissues. The inability of the kidney to produce erythropoietin affects the production of red blood cells and consequently can lead to anemia which will manifest in having shortness of breath especially on exertion or activity such as climbing the stairs or walking for long distances and you will also feel fatigued due to the lack of oxygen.

Since these symptoms manifest at a later stage, it is important to screen for kidney disease to detect diabetic nephropathy early on.

You can screen for diabetic nephropathy once a year. This is done by a simple test by providing a sample of your urine that will be tested for the presence of protein in the urine. Normally no protein is supposed to be present in the urine and the presence of protein in the urine is known as an indication of renal disease.

You will also be asked to provide a blood sample, and the blood sample will be able to detect the rate of glomerular filtration rate of your kidneys. This is an indication of how strong your kidneys are and how well they do their functions.

Your kidneys are one of the vital organs of your body and because nephropathy is a very common complication of diabetes, that is why it is very important to get yourself screened and tested at least once per year. The sooner you spot any emerging condition, the easier it can be treated.

Based on the test results the treatment will differ since there are five stages of kidney disease. The first 3 can be treated by a general practitioner and generally only require lifestyle modification and few medications, if anyat all. Stage 4 and 5 require you to be seen by a specialist as they need more advanced care.

Neuropathy

Diabetic neuropathy is a disorder involving the nerves which can be either sensory or motor or autonomic. Having diabetes type 1 or type 2 both pose a risk of developing diabetic neuropathy.

They can be categorized as either sensory neuropathy which affects the nerves that are responsible for sensory stimuli such as touch and temperature. In sensory neuropathy touch and temperature are affected, and it commonly presents in the feet and hands.

Motor neuropathy occurs to the motor nerves that are supplying the muscles and related to movements. Neuropathy in these nerves causes weakness.

Autonomic neuropathy affects the nerves which are responsible for involuntary actions such as heart rate, digestion and urination.

Being diabetic and poorly controlling it as well as being overweight with uncontrolled blood pressure and a bad lipid profiles plus being above 40 put you at risk of diabetic neuropathy. Neuropathy affects about 50% of the people in the diabetes population.

The symptoms of neuropathy can be numbness or pain in the hands, feet arms or legs and mostly in the periphery. However, diabetic neuropathy can also affect nerves supplying other organs such as the heart and sex organs causing erectile dysfunction.

The exact mechanism of how glucose damages the nervous system is still unknown, however it has been proven that the prolonged exposure to high amounts of glucose levels, damages the nerves and leading to the development of neuropathy with all its consequent effects. Having high levels of triglycerides, which is a type of fat, along with diabetes also increases your risk of developing nerve damage. Other factors such as vitamin B deficiency, smoking, having chronic liver disease or alcohol intake all increase your risk of developing diabetic neuropathy. Some anticancer medications are also associated with allowing neuropathy to develop.

In addition to the main symptoms of numbness, tingling and pain, you may start to feel wasting of your muscles in the feet and hand as well as weakness, unexplained diarrhea or constipation, sexual impotence, vaginal dryness, dizziness, urinary problems, nausea, vomiting etc.

If you start to suspect having diabetic neuropathy, perhaps it's time to head over for a physical exam. The doctor will check your reflexes, sensitivity, strength as well as other things. He may order other tests such as electromyography or nerve conduction studies to check the health of your nerves. If you have diabetes you are advised to have an annual exam for neuropathy especially if you're over 40.

Keeping your blood glucose levels under control and maintaining them is almost enough to prevent the development of this complication. In addition, certain diet, exercise and medication can promote the nerve health as well as control of uncontrolled hypertension and the correction of lipid profile can all help to prevent the development of diabetic neuropathy.

Certain targeted exercise can also be very effective in stimulating the circulation and strengthening the muscles. Having peripheral neuropathy can lead you to have numbness or weakness in your feet. Foot care is often emphasized for diabetics as there are several related complications that can occur. In fact, 1 out of 10 diabetics can develop small wounds or blisters that can be complicated with eventual amputation. When you have diabetic neuropathy, you may be unaware of any small ulcers or infections that occur on your foot and due to poor wound healing, ulcers or wounds will heal extremely slowly and may pose a greater risk for infection as they can get infected easily.

It should be one of your critical priorities to care for your feet. Check your feet regularly for any signs of foot ulcers, for example, any open wounds on the foot or any deformities or discoloration. Look for cuts, bruises, grazes, sores or swelling or any hard skin. Seek your doctor if you witness any of the above signs.

How does Eating High Carb Sugary Meals Increase Risk Factors Associated with Diabetes?

We mentioned earlier that diabetes type 2 is the cells inability to respond to insulin or the pancreatic cells not being able to produce enough insulin. So how does each of these conditions occur? For whatever reason, if your pancreas is not producing enough insulin and you continue to eat high carb sugary meals, the little insulin that was produced will not be able to drop the high blood glucose levels back to normal after meals.

As a result, the pancreas cells will still detect high blood glucose levels and will try to produce more and more insulin. However, the pancreas has a production capacity of a certain amount, but the constant stimulation causes it to try and exceed its production capacity of insulin. Eventually, this leads to the exhaustion of the pancreatic cells. When this happens after every meal that is loaded with sugars day after day, the pancreatic cells eventually wear out and can become permanently damaged. Though they mostly only become temporarily damaged and return to their normal state when the glucose stress subsides. That is why lowering blood glucose via eating a low carb diet or exercising is an effective strategy to reverse and manage diabetes type 2.

The second issue regarding eating high carb meals is that you are producing lots of insulin in order to be able to bring the glucose levels back to normal. The excessive exposure to insulin desensitizes the cells and makes them unresponsive to insulin.

When the cells lose their sensitivity to insulin, they become unable to respond to the signal of insulin that triggers cells to remove glucose from the blood. As a result, when the cells develop insulin insensitivity, no matter how much insulin is produced, the blood will still have increased levels of glucose. As a result, the pancreatic cells are still affecting high glucose levels and are trying to produce more and more insulin. As you see, this results in a vicious cycle, exhausting the pancreatic cells and increasing the insulin insensitivity of the cells. When your pancreatic cells are exhausted, you can no longer produce insulin, and if insulin is produced, it is produced in very low and insufficient amounts which further contributes to developing diabetes type 2. Following a low carb diet can help you decrease the risk of developing diabetes type 2.

How Having a Low Carb Diet Reduces the Risk of Developing Diabetes Type 2

When you minimize your intake of sugars and carbohydrates, you shift your metabolism into a healthier alternative that decreases your risk factors of developing diabetes type 2.

To begin with, having a reduced intake of carbohydrates and sugar means you decrease the body's need to release insulin in large quantities. This has a twofold benefit as it protects your pancreatic cells from exhaustion as they no longer need to secrete insulin in crazy amounts to restore your rising blood glucose levels. Moreover, it prevents insulin insensitivity from occurring as your cells are not exposed to large amounts of insulin frequently.

Other benefits of reducing your carb intake is that you are going to lose weight. Being overweight is a risk factor for developing diabetes. An additional fact is that too much insulin relates to weight gain.

Insulin in nature is an anabolic hormone. That means it causes the macromolecules to be built. Macromolecules are molecules such as fats and carbohydrates. So, in other words, insulin causes fats to be built rather than broken down, and this is the opposite of losing weight. This is in fact how you gain weight.

Additionally, your body uses mainly glucose for respiration. However, you can shift the molecule that your body uses for respiration and cause your body to burn fat rather than glucose. However, when there is an abundance of glucose available, your body will always be burning glucose and will leave fats alone.

Fat molecules in the presence of insulin, the anabolic hormone, will be built up and stored. This leads to the accumulation of fat around your organs and under your skin leaving you to gain weight overall. Weight gain further makes you lazy to exercise or carry on a physically active lifestyle, further increasing your risk of developing or worsening your diabetes.

The fats can also accumulate in your arteries and near your heart, leading you to have atherosclerosis, which is a condition that increases your risk of cardiovascular diseases and predisposes you to develop hypertension. So overall, simple and healthy habits such as having predominantly high carbohydrates and high in sugar diet can lead to a cascade of disorders including aggravating diabetes type 2 and increasing your risk of developing diabetes if you didn't have t; as well as increasing your risk of developing cardiac disorders.

How is Diabetes Diagnosed?

You can get checked by your doctor when you suspect having diabetes by noticing any of the previously mentioned symptoms as well as having one or more of the above-mentioned risk factors. You can hand over to your GP and request a blood glucose test. The lab technician will draw some blood from you. This can be a fasting test or a non-fasting test.

You can also have an oral glucose tolerance test in which you will have a fasting glucose test first and then you will be given a sugary drink and then having your blood glucose tested 2 hours after that to see how your body responds to glucose meals. In healthy individuals, the blood glucose should drop again 2 hours post sugary meals due to the action of insulin.

Another indicative test is the HbA1C. This test reflects the average of your blood glucose level over the last 2 to 3 months. It is also a test to see how well you manage your diabetes.

How Diabetes is Managed

People with diabetes type 1 require compulsory insulin shots to control their diabetes because they have no other option. People with diabetes type 2 can regulate their diabetes with healthy eating and regular physical activity although they may require some glucose-lowering medications that can be in tablet form or in the form of an injection.

All the above goes in the direction that you need to avoid a starchy diet because of its tendency to raise the blood glucose levels. Too many carbohydrates can lead to insulin sensitivity and pancreatic fatigue; as well as weight gain with all its associated risk factors for cardiovascular disease and hypertension. The solution is to lower your sugar intake, therefore, decrease your body's need for insulin and increase the burning of fat in your body.

When your body is low on sugars, it will be forced to use a subsequent molecule to burn for energy, in that case, this will be fat. The burning of fat will lead you to lose weight.

Understanding a Low Carb Diet

The definition of a low-carb diet is one that has very little carbohydrates. There are many types of low carb diets but the ones that proved to be beneficial to managing diabetes,substituted the carbs with a source of healthy fats. That way, it becomes a low carb, high-fat diet. If you are going to cut the carbs, you need to provide your body with an alternative source of energy. In this case, it is healthy fats.

That means greatly minimizing or cutting out foods that are high in starch and carbs such as rice, pasta, processed sugary foods, foods containing flour like white bread, etc. While loading up your diet with high fiber and low glycemic index foods such as vegetables, healthy fats and proteins to a lesser extent.

In addition to managing your diabetes, a low-carb diet is a healthy way to lose weight and promote your overall health. It converts your body from being a sugar burning machine into a fat burning machine. However, note that there is a transition period of about 7 to 14 days before your body successfully and completely switches from burning sugars to burning fats. During this transition period, your body will suffer from mild changes due to the deprivation of carbs (remember, it still depends on carbs during the transition period).

Problems with a Low Carb Diet

You will also be faced with initial fatigue from the shift in your diet and lowering your glucose intake. If you are type 1 diabetic, you need to be very careful about making dietary habit changes as this requires modification of your insulin dose which is why you need to consult your doctor before making any changes to your diet. The less carbohydrates you ingest, the less insulin you will need and therefore, you will not need the same amount of insulin dose as you used to take when you were having regular or high carb diet.

As your body transitions from a high carb state to a low carb state, you will be faced with some problems, but this should not discourage you. Here is a list of problems that you may face in the short transition period when you initially start a low-carb diet:

- You may start to feel lightheaded or dizzy, get headaches or feel fatigued but this will quickly go away within few days as your body starts to adapt to using fats for energy instead of sugars. If this problem persists or if it is affecting your normal daily functions, stop the low carb diet immediately and consult your doctor.

- You may find yourself having problems with retaining water as the carbohydrates help in water retention. When you decrease your carb intake, you will start to shed off more water than your body normally is used to lose. Loss of water is often accompanied with loss of salt; this may lead you to feel cramps or experience rapid heartbeats. You may also feel your pressure

59

drop due to the loss of water. You can compensate by drinking lots of water and adding minerals to it. These changes are only temporary and should subside after some time; however, if you remain feeling tired, dizzy or fatigued, consult your doctor immediately.

Aren't Fats Unhealthy?

We mentioned that it is important to include fat in replacement of the decreased carb intake. This raises the questions, aren't fats unhealthy? It is a misconception to assume that fat are unhealthy. In fact, they are an essential component in our body. Your body needs fats to synthesize many hormones and this goes into the composition of our cell membrane. Fats are also heat insulators, preserving your body's heat. They also lie around your vital organs, such as the kidney, protecting it from trauma. A moderate amount of fat is necessary for a healthy body. However, the problem with fats occurs when it exceeds the normal range.

There are healthy fats and unhealthy fats. The same goes for cholesterol. There is good cholesterol and bad cholesterol. Fish, olive oil and eggs, etc. contain natural fats. However, synthetic hydrogenated fats are considered an unhealthy type.

Good cholesterol is associated with HDL. It is a healthy and desirable type of cholesterol as it helps lower your lipids and improve your lipid profile. This contrasts with LDL which has undesirable health effects on your body. Therefore, it is important to distinguish between the different types of fats to know what foods to opt for and what foods to avoid

Examples of healthy fats include monounsaturated fats and polyunsaturated fats.

Examples of monounsaturated fats:

-   Avocados, olives, peanut butter, oils like sesame oil, peanut oil, canola oil, and olive oil

-   Nuts like peanuts, almonds, hazelnuts, pecans and cashews.

Examples of polyunsaturated fats:

-   Sunflower seeds, sesame seeds, and pumpkin seeds.

-   Nuts like walnuts.

-   Fatty fish like salmon, tuna, mackerel, sardines, and fish oil.

-   Plant oils like soya bean, and safflower oil.

-   Tofu, soya milk.

Examples of unhealthy fats includes trans fats and saturated fats.

Examples of trans fats:

-   All the commercially baked cookies, doughnuts, pastries, muffins, pizza dough, etc.

-   Packaged snacks such as microwave popcorn, chips, or crackers.

-   Hydrogenated margarine.

- Fried food such as fried chicken, chicken nuggets, breaded fish, French fries.

- Food that contains hydrogenated vegetable oils.

<u>Examples of saturated fats</u>:

- Chicken skin,

- Hydrogenated butter,

- Ice creams,

- Fatty meat.

General Habits to Decrease your Carb Intake

There are many ways to decrease your carb intake. Everything lies in the small habits, especially your shopping habits as that is where it all begins. When you are shopping, avoid items like bakeries in general and pastries as they are full of carbs. Instead, load up your shopping cart with vegetables. Did you know that you can have a 20 grams of carbs by either a plateful of assorted vegetables or a slice of bread? Guess which one makes you fuller and which one is healthier?

Start substituting main course items with healthy alternatives. For example, you can replace rice with cauliflower by grinding it in a blender to make cauliflower rice. It is almost the same and is much healthier.

You can also replace the pastries in your shopping cart with healthy alternatives such as meat, eggs, chicken, food that make you feel full while also loading up your body with healthy nutrients.

When you are shopping, avoid shopping for processed food or candy and sweets as they are full of artificial sweeteners as well as sugars that will cause you to exceed the physiological recommended carb limit with just a few bites.

Instead, you can opt-in for fruits. Fruits are like candy from nature; however, be careful to choose foods that have a low glycemic index such as avocados, strawberries, berries, peaches etc. Decrease your intake of fruits that have a high glycemic index such as bananas.

I am someone who loves sauces very much. It is very important for dipping and to flavor your food. Unfortunately, sauces like ketchup, barbecue sauce, maple syrup or even jam are full of sugars and sweeteners that are rich in carbs as well as artificial flavors. This can shoot up and skyrocket your blood glucose levels in just a few mouthfuls. Instead, you can have low carb healthy alternatives of dipping sauces such as pesto, seasoned tomato sauce, hummus, tahini, etc. You can also go for high fat options such as natural healthy butter, olive oil and coconut oil for salad dressings as well as mayonnaise.

Energy drinks, sports drinks and fizzy drinks are dangerous not only to your diet but your health too. If you love having fluids, it is a good option to blend some low glycemic fruits and make a smoothie to enjoy or drink plenty of water or skimmed milk. It is much healthier in terms of managing diabetes and in terms of promoting your overall health to drink fruit smoothies as they contain lots of nutrients and vitamins that are beneficial for your overall health. Sweetened tea, coffee with sugar, flavored coffee or chocolate drinks and energy drinks are some of the worst options you can have as they are full of sugars instead you can have black coffee with low fat milk.

Snacking can be one of the subconscious ways in which we load up on sugars without even realizing it. All those chips, crisps and crackers are full of artificial flavors as well as refined, processed sugars. A healthy option is to snack on celery or carrots. Snacking on cucumber bites with tahini sauce is a very healthy low carb snack option that is also full of fibers which is beneficial for your colon health and also helps lowering your cholesterol.

Meat, fish and seafood, chicken and eggs are proteins that are good for you. Keep the meat low fat. If you are eating poultry, trim the skin off. Moreover, it is better to go for plant-based protein as you will get more nutrients and fibers that are not present in animal products. Try to avoid fried meat or meat that has high fat cuts, for example, ribs, pork, bacon, added cheese or deep fried fish are all unhealthy options due to the added unhealthy fats.

Fats, oils and sweets are some of the favorite food of many people however you need to be extra careful about your choice of fats from natural sources for example vegetables and nuts seeds avocados are very healthy. However, try to keep to small proportions of foods that also give you Omega-3 fatty acids such as salmon, tuna and mackerel are also a healthy options in addition to grape seed oil, olive oil and l and plant-based oils. For healthy options try to avoid anything that has trans-fat in it and also avoid partially hydrogenated fats.

It can be hard in the beginning, but you have to skip on desserts such as ice cream and any sugar loaded food. You can keep those options as a reward on your cheat day. If you are craving a dessert, you can try dipping some of low glycemic index fruits in some heavy whipped cream or cream cheese while topping it off with berries. This is a very healthy way to stay low carb while also gaining fat which you need. If you absolutely must have chocolates, it is a much healthier option to go for dark chocolate, however, try not to do that often.

A Quick Introduction to the Glycemic Index

We mentioned snacking on low glycemic index fruits. So, let us elaborate on what that means. The glycemic index is a way to rank the carbohydrates based on their effects on the blood glucose levels in terms of how fast certain food raises blood glucose levels after intake. Foods with a lower glycemic index mean they are slow to cause a rise in the blood glucose levels. This effect can be different from one person to another. The general recommendation to people who have diabetes is to include high-fiber food that also has a low glycemic index, however, note that not all foods that are high in fiber have a low glycemic index.

Food that is considered having a low glycemic index are those with a GI less than 55. A glycemic index between 55 and 70 is considered intermediate. Foods with high glycemic index have a glycemic index larger than 70.

You can also alternate between eating low and intermediate glycemic index foods. It is not wise to completely exclude high glycemic index food. However, the rule is to minimize it.

General Guide when Choosing Food to Eat

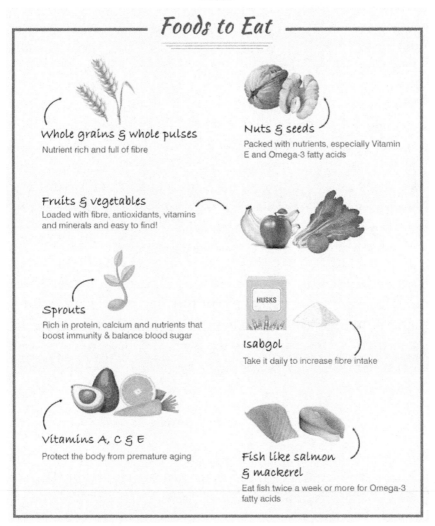

Foods to Eat

Whole grains & whole pulses
Nutrient rich and full of fibre

Nuts & seeds
Packed with nutrients, especially Vitamin E and Omega-3 fatty acids

Fruits & vegetables
Loaded with fibre, antioxidants, vitamins and minerals and easy to find!

Sprouts
Rich in protein, calcium and nutrients that boost immunity & balance blood sugar

HUSKS

Isabgol
Take it daily to increase fibre intake

Vitamins A, C & E
Protect the body from premature aging

Fish like salmon & mackerel
Eat fish twice a week or more for Omega-3 fatty acids

No matter what kind of diet you are attempting to follow, it is not correct to completely eliminate an entire food group. While in diabetes there are certain food groups that you can try to minimize your intake of such as starch and sugars but don't fall prey to the mistake of completely eliminating starch as your body needs carbs. Instead, what you must do is to choose wisely between the various food options in each category to ensure that you ingest the best and most suitable food type from each category and avoid the ones that will worsen your condition.

The goal of controlling your food with diabetes is eating food that will not increase your blood glucose levels higher than normal. At the same time it needs to be food that makes you feel full and keeps hunger at bay; in addition, certain food categories can promote your health and provide you with nutritional elements that can help you fight off diabetes and protect you from its complications.

It is important to note that there is no one-size-fits-all when it comes to healthy eating plans for diabetic patients. There are lots of personal variations in the way our body responds tonutrition and different food intake styles however there are general rules that can be observed if you have diabetes and wish to control your blood sugar and keep its complications at bay.

Low Starch Food

Whole grains for example, oatmeal, quinoa and brown rice are preferred and healthier than white rice, white flour or processed grains, macaroni, etc.

Baked sweet potato provides a low carb option in contrast to regular potato such as French fries. Other items that contain high carbs include white bread and white flour etc. Instead, opt for whole grain foods that have very little added sugar or not at all.

Non-Starchy Vegetables

One of the healthiest options if you're diabetic is to include a couple of servings of non-starchy vegetables per day. There is very little chance that you could go wrong with overeating non-starchy vegetables, that is because they have a very low calorific intake.

Non starchy vegetables are vegetables that contain a small amount of carbohydrate. This is typically about 5 grams or less of carbohydrate per a 100g of serving. It is recommended by the American Diabetes Association that you have your plate half-filled with non-starchy vegetables.

Throughout your day, it should be your goal that you have at least five portions of fruit and vegetables and out of those 5, it is best to have at least three of them that are non-starchy vegetables.

There are several reasons why non-starchy vegetables are a very healthy options for diabetics. The foremost reason is that they are very low in carbs. Other reasons include how non-starchy vegetables are very nutritious. They are full of vitamins and minerals as well as other critical nutrients such as phytochemicals. In addition, being vegetables, they are a critical source of dietary fiber. The dietary fiber will help you to digest food properly and it also plays an important role in lowering your cholesterol levels. Overall, dietary fiber is an essential nutrient to include in your diet.

Non-starchy vegetables are a very powerful defense against the complications of diabetes. They help to protect your cells from the damage induced by the disorder of diabetes and promote the health of your blood vessels which can also be compromised during the course of diabetes progression.

Non-starchy vegetables are also rich in vitamins and minerals such as vitamin A, vitamin C and vitamin K. Vitamin C helps to promote your immunity and protect your cells from oxidative damage.

A good source of non-starchy vegetables containing vitamin C are peppers, sprouts and broccoli. You can easily add peppers to your salad or main dish. Steamed broccoli is also a very healthy option to add to your main dish or serve alongside salmon or to add to your veggie pan salad.

Vitamin E is also helpful in boosting your immune system; it is also important for your eye health as well as for your skin. Carrots, kale and spinach are options rich in vitamin E that you can easily add them to your food.

Vitamin K is going to assist in wound healing and improving health as well as preventing atherosclerosis. Diabetics are at risk of atherosclerosis if they have uncontrolled diabetes. Moreover, they have poor wound healing so food rich in vitamin K such as green leafy vegetables will help promote the health of diabetics and prevent infections as a result of poor wound healing.

Below are Some Examples of Non-Starchy Vegetables

Leafy vegetables: kale, lettuce, spinach, watercress, cabbage, Brussel sprouts.

Root vegetables: carrot, turnip, radishes.

Squashes: cucumber, squash, courgette, pumpkin.

Stalk vegetables: asparagus, leeks, spring onions, celery.

Others: broccoli, bean sprouts, mushroom, cauliflower, peppers, tomato.

As a diabetic, vegetables are your best friend. Fresh vegetables when eaten raw or even when steamed, roasted or grilled, can be a very healthy low carb option. The same applies to frozen vegetables that are lightly steamed. Always opt for low sodium or unsalted canned vegetables. Canned vegetables with lots of added sodium are not a healthy option.

Also, it is counterproductive if you eat veggies that are cooked with lots of butter cheese or a high carb source. If you are having hypertension or other complications of diabetes and metabolic syndrome then you need to limit your intake of sodium and that includes limiting pickles etc.

Fatty Fish

Examples: Herring, Salmon anchovies, mackerel, sardine.

Fatty fish are one of the most consistent diet recommendations when it comes to fending off diseases. Diabetes is no exception. Fish is one of the most beneficial foods you can eat if you have diabetes.

Since having diabetes poses a risk on your heart functions it is important to take cardioprotective measures. Salmon contains Omega-3 fatty acids which have a profound positive effect on your heart health. Taking care and promoting your heart health helps against the increased risk of heart disease and stroke that people with diabetes are faced with. In addition, studies have shown that several inflammatory markers had dropped when fatty fish was consumed 5 to 7 days per week for about 8 weeks. In addition to all that it contains high quality protein and is low in carbs, therefore, is perfect for maintaining normal blood glucose sugars after meals.

Dairy

Dairy food is an important food category and with a variety of choices available for you to pick from. Studies have shown that milk product consumption and total dairy products have been associated with a reduced risk of developing type 2 diabetes. It is also protective for those who have prediabetes. The mechanisms explaining this evidence is complicated but simply put, certain biomarker fatty acids found in dairy milk are associated with lowering the risk of developing diabetes type 2. The studies were conducted on each of the following items from the dairy group including whole milk and yoghurt in addition to total dairy consumption.

Examples of dairy food include milk, yoghurt, cream, butter and cheese. Unsweetened dairy products can be a very healthy choice for those who wish to follow a low-carb diet. There are numerous benefits for dairy foods as they are a good source of protein, calcium and vitamin B12. It is recommended by the National Osteoporosis Society that a daily intake of 700 mg of calcium is required for adults to maintain healthy bones as well as other functions that depend on calcium.

Vitamin B12 is an important source for the nervous system. Diabetics are at risk of complications of neuropathy that affects the peripheral nerves. Vitamin B12 helps protect against some of the complications of diabetes concerning the nerves. The protein in milk is also important for muscle repair and growth. The recommended daily intake of calcium can be achieved by just a pint of milk along with another source that includes food such as beans, fish with edible bones such as sardines and salmon and dark green vegetables, for example, kale and broccoli.

For dairy opt for low-fat dairy if you want to have high fat or full fat dairy do so but in small proportions. The best choices are skimmed milk, low-fat yoghurt and low-fat or non-fat sour cream or cottage cheese. Some of the worst choices are whole milk, regular yoghurt, regular sour cream, cottage cheese and ice cream etc.

Beans and Pulses

Beans, pulses: lentils peas chickpeas and runner beans are all examples of non-animal sources of protein that can be very beneficial for diabetics.

Soya Beans have been included among this group and it has been supported with research indicating that the consumption of soya beans increases insulin sensitivity and reduces the risk of developing type 2 diabetes. In fact, certain countries in Asia have been using black soya beans to combat type 2 diabetes.

Adding beans to your salads is a good option for increasing your protein intake.

Fruits

Just like vegetables, fruits are one of the healthiest food groups that you can add to your diet. They are rich in nutrients especially vitamin Cwhich helps to keep your cells healthy. In addition to the minerals, we also have fiber which help digestion, and it reduces cholesterol levels. Different fruits have a different combination of vitamins and minerals; for example, grapefruits can be rich in vitamin A as well as potassium; they can also be rich in vitamin K and manganese. A meta-analysis showed that groups of people who consumed higher amount of fruits were at less risk of developing type 2 diabetes.

It is recommended by the American Diabetes Association to use fruits as a dessert option rather than having a sugar-loaded desserts such as ice cream. While fruits have dense nutrients as well as fiber and antioxidants it is important to remember that certain foods have a high glycemic index and can increase your blood sugar levels, therefore, it is important to be mindful about the types of fruits you eat and when.

Bananas and oranges are fruits that have high glycemic index while berries for example or less sugary.

Below are some examples of <u>fruits that have a glycemic index of under 55</u>:

Grapefruit, grapes, kiwi, apples, avocados, peaches, plums strawberries.

Fruit with medium glycemic index from 56 to 69:

Pineapples, papayas, honeydew melon.

Foods with high glycemic index that is more than 70:

Watermelon and dates.

Avoid processed foods such as apple sauce that have had their fiber removed. if you have a sweet tooth, fruits can be an optimum way to satisfy your desires without compromising your health. Since fruits are high in nutrients and low in fat and sodium, they are optimum if you have obesity or hypertension.

One serving of fruit is a medium-sized fruit that is the size of the piece. Or or a cup ofsmaller fruits such as berries. So, you should avoid it, but if you have processed fruits have only half a cup of processed fruits to fulfil the serving size.

Apples. An apple is a versatile fruit that you can snack on raw or cook it with some flavoring such as cinnamon or ginger to make a delicious dessert. You can also stuff your apples with some crushed nuts such as walnuts or pecans.

Avocados. Avocado's are very high in healthy fats which are the Mono- unsaturated fats that are beneficial to your body. Avocados are a tasty option to add to your main dish; slice along with some salmon or make guacamole. They're very easy to prepare or include in any of your dishes.

Berries. Berries are a very delicious and versatile fruit. There are strawberries, blueberries, blackberries, etc. There are a lot of things that you can do with berries, for example, you can eat them raw or you can make them into a smoothie.

You can always add various berries to most of your breakfast or snacks, for example, making an oatmeal breakfast or adding various to your fresh whipped cream or frozen yoghurt. They are also rich in antioxidants and very low on calories. They help fight inflammation and other diseases such as cancer.

Citrus fruits. They are also good for boosting your immunity; they are loaded with vitamin C.One orange contains all the amount of vitamin c that you require in a day. Since immunity is an issue with diabetics adding citrus foods to your diet is very healthy and useful low carb option. You can add lemons to your seafood or sauces or even to your iced water or tea. You can simply make lemons or oranges into a refreshing cold drink. The folate and potassium in oranges help you to equalize your blood pressure if you suffer from hypertension. Citrus foods also include grapefruits as well as oranges and lemons.

Peaches. They are juicy and delicious fragrant foods that contain lots of nutrients such as vitamins A and C as well as fiber and minerals such as potassium. They are easy to add in your yoghurt or spice them up with some cinnamon or ginger. You can also flavor your tea with peach instead of sugar for a healthy twist on your drinks.

Pears. They are also a tasty treat that you can add up to your salad or snack on. They are rich in fiber and are a good source of vitamin K.

Kiwi is a slightly citrus fruit that is rich in fiber and vitamin C as well as potassium. One large kiwi contains about 13 grams of carbohydrates which is low carb, making it a delicious yet very healthy option to add to your diet.

Lean Meat

A source of protein that is low in fat and low in calorie is lean meat. That means the red meat such as pork chops that are trimmed of fat or skinless chicken or turkey.

A nutritional source of protein for promoting cell health and repair is lean meat while also being a low carb and low-fat option. Poultry is also a rich source of vitamin B3, B6 choline and selenium. Vitamin B3 which is known as niacin helps with stress and sex hormones. Erectile dysfunction and stress are an issue for those who have diabetes and having food with vitamin B3 become very beneficial for diabetics. Niacin helps with promoting the function of nerves and can reduce inflammation. Selenium has strong antioxidant properties that help with controlling inflammation and protecting the cells. Selenium also has a function in promoting the immune system which is very beneficial for people with diabetes.

Red meat is also a rich source of protein, iron, zinc and vitamin B. Iron is important for your red blood cells,to transport oxygen, as healthy cells require a constant supply of oxygen. Anemia which is a deficiency in RBCs can occur due to a deficiency in iron which is a condition that could easily be avoided by eating adequate amounts of iron. Iron can also be found in dark green leafy plants, as well as beans, iron from greens is the best source.

Zinc is also a mineral needed by the body for the synthesis of DNA. It also has a role in helping the immune system to function properly. You can also find zinc in fish eggs as well as beans, although zinc is better absorbed from fish and meat sources.

Red meat is rich in vitamin B6 and B12. Both are helpful for promoting the immune system,regeneration and protection of the nervous system. One medication that some diabetics take is known as metformin causes an increased drop in vitamin B12. Therefore, it becomes necessary to compensate for the loss of vitamin B from sources such as red meat.

Eggs

Be mindful about the number of eggs you consume as they can easily raise your cholesterol levels. If you're going to eat an egg, it is preferred that it's boiled and consume the whole egg as the benefits of eggs lines in the nutrients inside,rather than the whites. It is a debate whether eggs are helpful or not for diabetics due to due to their low carb content; however, consuming an excessive amount of eggs is associated with the risk of increasing cholesterol levels. Moreover, apart from being rich in cholesterol, eggs are dense in nutrients as they have essential fatty acids proteins and vitamin D.

Nuts

Studies have found that nuts help to decrease the risk of developing type 2 diabetes the *Journal of the American College of Nutrition* stated that consumption of nuts is associated with decreasing the prevalence of certain risk factors that are associated with developing type 2 diabetes and other metabolic disorders. Some have more benefits than other, for example, almonds are rich in nutrients particularly vitamin E. Cashews contain a lot of magnesium.

Almonds, cashews and peanuts are nuts that help to reduce the bad cholesterol. Walnuts are rich in Omega-3 fatty acids

Nuts that work on reducing the bad cholesterol are very effective because they protect diabetics from the complication of the narrowing of arteries.

Cashews. Consuming cashews is very beneficial to lower your blood pressure and decrease the risk of heart disease and therefore reduce the risk of gettingdiabetes type 2. They are also low in calories; therefore, they have no negative effect on your blood glucose level. They are also low in fat, so they do not affect your weight negatively. You can have about a handful of cashews every day for the maximum benefit.

Peanuts. Peanuts are rich in fiber and protein, and therefore they are a beneficial option for people suffering from diabetes. You can have up to 25 to 30 peanuts every day. You can also roast them. They have the ability to control your blood glucose levels.

Pistachios. They are loaded with energy however they are good sources of protein and a good source of healthy fats which can make you feel full for a long time, therefore, curbing the urge to snack. A study performed showed that eating pistachios was very beneficial for people suffering from diabetes. Avoid salted pistachios however.

Walnuts are high in calories; however, they do not affect your body weight. They have numerous nutritional benefits and consuming walnuts daily can help in weight loss due to their low carbohydrate content and their possession of substances that activate the fat burning pathways. They also educe fasting glucose, which help you avoid obesity as a complication of diabetes. The high calorie content helps your body by providing it with energy so that you don't feel like eating a lot and therefore gain weight.

Almonds control the blood glucose level and are very beneficial for diabetics because they help to reduce the oxidative stress which affects cells in diabetics. They are also rich in magnesium. Avoid salted almonds, and you can also soak them in water overnight to eat them fresh the next day.

Foods to Avoid

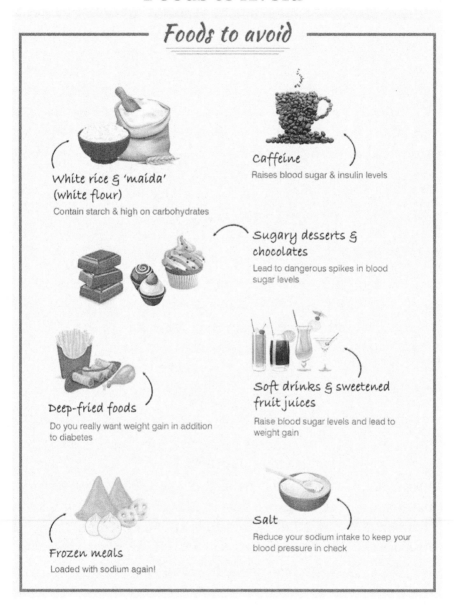

Foods to avoid

White rice & 'maida' (white flour)
Contain starch & high on carbohydrates

Caffeine
Raises blood sugar & insulin levels

Sugary desserts & chocolates
Lead to dangerous spikes in blood sugar levels

Deep-fried foods
Do you really want weight gain in addition to diabetes

Soft drinks & sweetened fruit juices
Raise blood sugar levels and lead to weight gain

Frozen meals
Loaded with sodium again!

Salt
Reduce your sodium intake to keep your blood pressure in check

Beverages that are sweetened with sugar

These beverages are some of the worst choices to obtain for diabetics. This is because they are very high in carbs. For example, a 12 oz can of soda has roughly 38 grams of carbs. The same applies for sweetened iced tea or sweetened lemonade as they contain about 35 g of carbs per serving.

Moreover, these sweetened drinks are full of fructose which has been strongly associated with increased insulin resistance and worsening of diabetes. On top of promoting diabetes, high levels of fructose also results in having belly fat and leads to the build-up of harmful cholesterol and increases the level of triglycerides. This shift in metabolism will not help to control your diabetes.

Trans fats

These are fats that are made by adding hydrogen to unsaturated fatty acids in order to stabilize them. Examples of trans fats can be found in margarine and frozen dinners. In addition, many food companies add trans fats to the muffins and baked goods to give them a better taste and extend their expiry date.

Trans fats do not have a direct effect on raising your blood glucose levels, however, they increase your insulin resistance and promote the accumulation of fat. Don't disturb your fat metabolism and decrease your good cholesterol, because this has an indirect effect on losing control of managing your diabetes. Also, since diabetics have an increased risk of heart disease, all the above actions of trans fats further increase the risk of developing heart disease.

Pasta, rice and white bread

All these foods are rich in carbohydrates and quickly get digested to release lots of glucose into the blood. A study has shown that ingesting a meal consisting of a high-carb bagels resulted in significantly raising the blood glucose levels as well as decreasing the brain function in people who have type 2 diabetes. In addition, these foods are low in nutrients and have very little fiber so the overall nutritional value is almost insignificant. Food rich in fiber is important for controlling diabetes, your cholesterol levels and blood pressure and therefore the main bulk of your food should be dedicated to foods that are high in fiber.

Fruit flavored yoghurt

Simple plain yoghurt is a very healthy option for diabetics. On the contrary, yoghurt that is fruit flavored is completely different. They are often made from non-fat milk and they are loaded with carbohydrates and sugars. In fact, one serving of fruit flavored yoghurt has about 47 grams of carbohydrates in the form of sugar. Instead of choosing yogurt that is flavored and rich in sugars, opt for simple whole milk yoghurt that is free of sugar and helpful for your gut health as well as helpful to lose weight.

There are also some fruits to avoid overeating if you are diabetic.

Grapes

A single grape contains 1 gram of carbohydrates that means if you eat 30 grapes, you have easily eaten 30g of carbs. And you can eat the same number of berries or strawberries while having significantly less amount of carbohydrates.

Cherries

They are super delicious that is why it is hard to stop eating them once you have started, however, they are very rich in sugars and can cause your blood sugar to spike quickly.

Pineapple

When fresh and ripe, they can have a very high glycemic index. If you must eat pineapples try to have a small serving of about half a cup and eat it with food that is low-fat, for example, Greek yoghurt. Don't eat canned pineapple as they are sweetened with unhealthy sugars.

Mango

These are super delicious foods, however one single mango has about 30 grams of carbohydrates and about 25 grams of sugars. A riper and softer mango will have a higher glycemic index, while mango that is firm will have a lower glycemic index relatively.

Banana

It is one of those too sweet, yet very delicious foods. A medium sized banana has about the same grams of carbohydrates that is double of any other fruit.

If you must have a banana try to have half a serving and refrigerate the rest of it for another time.

Dried fruits seem harmless, especially when you add them to your food, however, two tablespoons of dried raisins have a similar amount of carbohydrates as just one cup of blueberries or another small piece of another fruit. That is because the water content has dried out and their sugars have been greatly concentrated. Remove dried fruits from your diet and add fresh ones to your diet instead.

Diabetic Plate Recipes

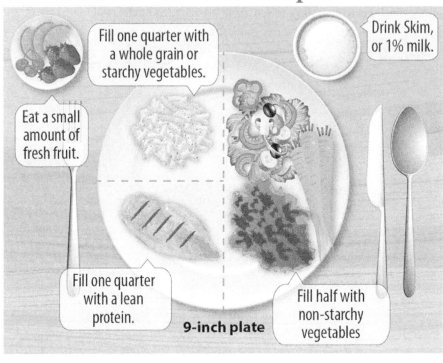

Chicken and Turkey Recipes

Pumpkin, Bean, and Chicken Enchiladas

Prep time: 35 minutes	Cook time: 25 minutes	Servings: 4

Ingredients

- o   Olive oil – 2 tsps.

- o   Chopped onion – ½ cup

- o   Jalapeno – 1, seeded and chopped

- o   Pumpkin – 1 (15 oz.) can

- o   Water – 1 ½ cups, more if needed

- o   Chili powder – 1 tsp.

- o   Salt – ½ tsp.

- o   Ground cumin – ½ tsp.

- o   Canned no-salt-added red kidney beans – 1 cup, rinsed and drained

- o   Shredded cooked chicken breast – 1 ½ cups

- o   Shredded part-skim mozzarella cheese – ½ cup

- o   Whole wheat tortillas – 8 (6-inch), softened

- o   Salsa and lime wedges

Method

1. Lightly coat a 2-qt. rectangular baking dish with cooking spray and preheat the oven to 400F.
2. In a saucepan, heat oil over medium heat. Add jalapeno and onion and stir-fry until onion is tender, for about 5 minutes. Stir in cumin, salt, chili powder, 1 ½ cups water and pumpkin and heat through. Add more water if needed.
3. Place beans in a bowl and mash slightly with a fork. Stir in ¼ cup of the cheese, the chicken, and half of the pumpkin mixture.
4. Spoon 1/3 cup bean mixture onto each tortilla. Roll up tortillas. Place in the baking dish (seam sides down). Pour remaining pumpkin mixture over enchiladas.
5. Bake, covered, for 15 minutes. Sprinkle with remaining ¼-cup cheese. Bake, uncovered until heated through, for about 10 minutes more.
6. Serve with salsa and lime wedges.

Nutritional Facts Per Serving (2 enchiladas each)

o   Calories: 357

o   Fat: 8g

o   Carb: 44g

o   Protein: 28g

Mu Shu Chicken

Prep time: 20 minutes	Cook time: 6 hours	Servings: 6

Ingredients

- Hoisin sauce – ½ cup
- Water – 2 Tbsp.
- Toasted sesame oil - 4 tsp.
- Cornstarch – 1 Tbsp.
- Reduced-sodium soy sauce – 1 Tbsp.
- Garlic – 3 cloves, minced
- Shredded cabbage with carrots – 1 (16-oz.) pkg. (coleslaw mix)
- Coarsely shredded carrots – 1 cup
- Skinless, boneless chicken thighs – 12 oz.
- Whole wheat flour tortillas – 6 (8-inch)
- Green onions

Method

1. Combine the first six ingredients in a bowl (through garlic).
2. In a slow cooker, combine shredded carrots and coleslaw mix.

3. Cut chicken into 1/8 inch slices, cut each slice in half lengthwise. Place chicken on top of the cabbage mix. Drizzle with ¼ cup of the hoisin mixture.
4. Heat tortillas according to package directions. Fill tortillas with chicken mixture.
5. Top with green onions and serve.

Nutritional Facts Per Serving

o Calories: 269

o Fat: 8g

o Carb: 34g

o Protein: 16g

Stove-Top Chicken, Macaroni, and Cheese

Prep time: 10 minutes	Cook time: 30 minutes	Servings: 5

Ingredients

- Dried multigrain or elbow macaroni – 1 ½ cups
- Skinless, boneless chicken breast halves – 12 oz. cut into 1-inch pieces
- Chopped onion – ¼ cup
- Light semisoft cheese with garlic and fine herbs – 1 (6.5 oz.) pkg.
- Fat-free milk – 1 2/3 cups
- All-purpose flour – 1 Tbsp.
- Shredded reduced-fat cheddar cheese – ¾ cup
- Fresh baby spinach – 2 cups
- Cherry tomatoes – 1 cup, quartered

Method

1. Cook macaroni according to package directions. Drain.
2. Meanwhile, coat a skillet with cooking spray. Heat skillet over medium high heat.
3. Add onion and chicken until chicken is no longer pink, about 4 to 6 minutes. Stirring frequently.

Remove from heat and stir in semisoft cheese until melted.

4. In a bowl, whisk together flour and milk until smooth. Gradually stir milk mixture into chicken mixture. Cook and stir until bubbly and thickened. Lower heat and gradually add cheddar cheese. Stirring until melted.

5. Add cooked macaroni, cook and stir for 1 to 2 minutes or until heated through.

6. Stir in spinach. Top with cherry tomatoes and serve.

Nutritional Facts Per Serving

o   Calories: 369

o   Fat: 12g

o   Carb: 33g

o   Protein: 33g

Chicken Sausage Omelets with Spinach

Prep time: 20 minutes	Cook time: 10 minutes	Servings: 2

Ingredients

- Fresh spinach – 2 cups

- Frozen fully cooked chicken and maple breakfast sausage links – ½ of a 7-oz. pkg. thawed and chopped

- Eggs – 3, lightly beaten

- Water – 2 Tbsp.

- Shredded part-skim mozzarella cheese – ¼ cup

- Green onions – 2, green tops only, thinly sliced

- Grape tomatoes – ½ cup, quartered

- Fresh basil leaves – ¼ cup, thinly sliced

Method

1. Coat a skillet with nonstick cooking spray. Heat over medium heat.
2. Add sausage and spinach. Cook until sausage is heated. Remove from the skillet.
3. In a bowl, whisk together the water and eggs. Add egg mixture to skillet and cook until egg is set and shiny.
4. Spoon spinach and sausage mixture over half of the omelet. Sprinkle with cheese and green onions. Fold the opposite side of omelet over sausage mixture.

5. Cook for 1 minute or until filling is heated and cheese is melted.
6. Transfer to a plate and cut in half. Transfer half of the omelet to a second plate.
7. Top with tomatoes and basil and serve.

Nutritional Facts Per Serving

- o Calories: 252

- o Fat: 16g

- o Carb: 5g

- o Protein: 21g

Chicken-Broccoli Salad with Buttermilk Dressing

Prep time: 20 minutes	Cook time: 0 minutes	Servings: 4

Ingredients

- o Packaged shredded broccoli slaw mix – 3 cups
- o Coarsely chopped cooked chicken breast – 2 cups
- o Dried cherries – ½ cup
- o Sliced celery – 1/3 cup
- o Chopped red onion – ¼ cup
- o Buttermilk – 1/3 cup
- o Light mayonnaise – 1/3 cup
- o Honey – 1 Tbsp.
- o Cider vinegar – 1 Tbsp.
- o Dry mustard – 1 tsp.
- o Salt – ½ tsp.
- o Black pepper – 1/8 tsp.
- o Fresh baby spinach – 4 cups

Method

1. Combine the first five ingredients in a bowl (through onion). In a small bowl, whisk together the next seven

ingredients (through pepper). Pour buttermilk mixture over broccoli mixture. Toss to gently mix.

2. Cover and chill for 2 hours to 24 hours.
3. Add baby spinach and serve.

Nutritional Facts Per Serving

o   Calories: 278

o   Fat: 7g

o   Carb: 29g

o   Protein: 26g

Country-Style Wedge Salad with Turkey

Prep time: 10 minutes	Cook time: 0 minutes	Servings: 4

Ingredients

- Bibb or butterhead lettuce – 1 head, quartered
- Buttermilk-Avocado dressing – 1 recipe (see below)
- Shredded cooked turkey breast – 2 cups
- Halved grape or cherry tomatoes – 1 cup
- Hard-cooked eggs – 2, chopped
- Low-sodium, less-fat bacon – 4 slices, crisp-cooked, and crumbled
- Finely chopped red onion – ¼ cup
- Cracked black pepper

Method

1. Arrange one lettuce quarter on each plate. Drizzle half of the dressing over wedges. Top with turkey, eggs, and tomatoes. Drizzle with the remaining dressing. Sprinkle with onion, bacon and pepper.
2. To make the buttermilk-avocado dressing: in a blender, combine ¾ cup buttermilk, ½ avocado, 1 tbsp. parsley, ¼ tsp. each salt, onion powder, dry mustard, and black pepper, and 1 garlic clove, minced. Cover and blend until smooth.

Nutritional Facts Per Serving

- o   Calories: 228

- o   Fat: 9g

- o   Carb: 8g

- o   Protein: 29g

Turkey Kabob Pitas

Prep time: 25 minutes	Cook time: 15 minutes	Servings: 4

Ingredients

- Whole cumin seeds – 1 tsp. lightly crushed
- Shredded cucumber – 1 cup
- Seeded and chopped Roma tomato – 1/3 cup
- Slivered red onion – ¼ cup
- Shredded radishes – ¼ cup
- Snipped fresh cilantro – ¼ cup
- Black pepper – ¼ tsp.
- Turkey breast - 1 lb. cut into thin strips
- Curry blend – 1 recipe
- Plain fat-free Greek yogurt – ¼ cup
- Whole wheat pita bread rounds – 4 (6-inch)

Method

1. Soak wooden skewers in water for 30 minutes. Toast the cumin seeds for 1 minute and transfer to a bowl. Add the next six ingredients to the bowl (through pepper). Mix.

2. In another bowl, combine curry blend and turkey. Stir to coat. Thread turkey onto skewers.

3. Grill kabobs, uncovered for 6 to 8 minutes or until turkey is no longer pink. Turning kabobs occasionally.

4. Remove turkey from skewers. Spread Greek yogurt on pita breads. Spoon cucumber mixture over yogurt. Top with grilled turkey.

5. Serve.

To make the curry blend

1. In a bowl, combine 2 tsp. olive oil, 1 tsp. curry powder, ½ tsp, each ground turmeric, ground cumin, and ground coriander, ¼ tsp. ground ginger, and 1/8 tsp. salt and cayenne pepper.

Nutritional Facts Per Serving

o Calories: 343

o Fat: 6g

o Carb: 40g

o Protein: 35g

Beef and Lamb Recipes

Spicy Beef Sloppy Joes

Prep time: 20 minutes	Cook time: 8 hours	Servings: 12

Ingredients

- o   Lean ground beef – 2 lb.

- o   Lower-sodium salsa – 2 ½ cups

- o   Coarsely chopped fresh mushrooms – 3 cups

- o   Shredded carrots – 1 ¼ cups

- o   Finely chopped red and green sweet peppers – 1 ¼ cups

- o   No-salt added tomato paste – ½ (6-oz.) can

- o   Garlic – 4 cloves, minced

- o   Dried basil – 1 tsp. crushed

- o   Salt – ¾ tsp.

- o   Dried oregano – ½ tsp. crushed

- o   Cayenne pepper – ¼ tsp.

- o   Whole wheat hamburger buns – 12, split and toasted

Method

1. Cook ground beef in a skillet until browned. Drain off fat.
2. In a slow cooker, add the meat and combine the next 10 ingredients (through cayenne pepper).
3. Cover and cook on low for 8 to 10 hours or on high for 4 to 5 hours.
4. Spoon ½-cup of the meat mixture onto each bun.
5. Serve.

Nutritional Facts Per Serving

- Calories: 278

- Fat: 8g

- Carb: 29g

- Protein: 20g

Roasted Steak and Tomato Salad

Prep time: 20 minutes	Cook time: 20 minutes	Servings: 4

Ingredients

- Beef tenderloin steaks – 2 (8 oz.), trimmed
- Cracked black pepper – 1 tsp.
- Kosher salt – ¼ tsp.
- Small tomatoes – 6, halved
- Olive oil – 2 tsps.
- Shredded Parmesan cheese – ¼ cup
- Dried oregano – ½ tsp. crushed
- Torn romaine lettuce – 8 cups
- Artichoke hearts – 1 (14-oz.) can, drained and quartered
- Red onion slivers – 1/3 cup
- Balsamic vinegar – 3 Tbsp.
- Olive oil – 1 Tbsp.

Method

1. Preheat the oven to 400F.
2. Season the meat with salt and pepper and rub. Let stand for 20 minutes at room temperature.

3. Arrange tomato halves on a baking sheet (cut side down).
4. Heat 2 tsps. oil in a skillet. Add meat and cook until well browned on all sides, about 8 minutes. Transfer meat to other side of baking sheet.
5. Roast for 8 to 10 minutes for medium (145F). Remove meat from oven. Cover with foil and let stand. Move oven rack for broiling.
6. Turn oven to broil. Turn tomatoes cut sides up. Combine oregano and Parmesan. Sprinkle over tomatoes. Broil 4 to 5 inches from heat for about 2 minutes, or until cheese is melted and golden.
7. In a bowl, combine onion, artichoke hearts, and lettuce. Drizzle with vinegar and 1 tbsp. oil. Toss to coat.
8. Arrange on plates. Slice steak and arrange over lettuce with tomato halves.

Nutritional Facts Per Serving

o Calories: 299

o Fat: 14g

o Carb: 16g

o Protein: 29g

Lamb Fatteh with Asparagus

Prep time: 10 minutes	Cook time: 20 minutes	Servings: 4

Ingredients

- o Olive oil – 1 Tbsp.
- o Medium onion – 1, sliced
- o Garlic – 4 cloves, minced
- o Boneless lamb leg – 12 oz. cut into smaller pieces
- o 50% less sodium beef broth – 1 (14.5 oz.) can
- o Whole wheat pearl couscous - 1 cup
- o Dried oregano – ½ tsp. crushed
- o Ground cumin – ½ tsp.
- o Salt – ¼ tsp.
- o Black pepper – ¼ tsp.
- o Thin asparagus spears – 1 lb. sliced into 2-inch pieces
- o Chopped red sweet pepper – ¾ cup
- o Snipped fresh oregano and lemon wedges

Method

1. Heat oil in a skillet. Add onion and cook for 3 minutes.
2. Add garlic and cook for 1 minute.

3. Add lamb and cook until browned on all sides, about 3 to 5 minutes.
4. Stir in the next six ingredients (through black pepper). Bring to a boil. Lower heat and simmer, covered, for 10 minutes. Stirring occasionally.
5. Stir in sweet pepper and asparagus. Cover and simmer until vegetables are crisp-tender, about 3 to 5 minutes.
6. Fluff lamb mixture lightly with a fork. Top with fresh oregano.
7. Serve with lemon wedges.

Nutritional Facts Per Serving

o   Calories: 334

o   Fat: 9g

o   Carb: 39g

o   Protein: 26g

Prep time: 30 minutes	Cook time: 20 minutes	Servings: 4

Ingredients

- Boneless beef top sirloin steak – 6 oz.
- Olive oil – 1 tsp.
- Chopped onion – ½ cup
- Water – 2 cups
- Beef broth – 1 (14.5 oz.) can
- No-salt-added diced tomatoes – 1 (14.5 oz.) can, undrained
- Thinly sliced carrot – ½ cup
- Unsweetened cocoa powder – 1 tsp.
- Garlic – 1 clove, minced
- Thinly sliced cabbage – 1 cup
- Dried wide noodles – ½ cup
- Paprika – 2 tsps.
- Light sour cream – ¼ cup
- Snipped fresh parsley

Method

1. Cut meat into ½-inch cubes. In a saucepan, cook and stir meat in hot oil until browned, for about 6 minutes. Add onion, cook and stir until onion softens, about 3 minutes.
2. Stir in the next six ingredients (through garlic). Bring to a boil. Reduce heat. Simmer, uncovered, for about 15 minutes or until meat is tender.
3. Stir in paprika, noodles, and cabbage. Simmer, uncovered, until noodles are tender but still firm, for about 5 to 7 minutes. Remove from heat.
4. Top each serving with sour cream.
5. Sprinkle with parsley and additional paprika.
6. Serve.

Nutritional Facts Per Serving

o   Calories: 188

o   Fat: 7g

o   Carb: 16g

o   Protein: 14g

Beef-Vegetable Ragout

Prep time: 30 minutes	Cook time: 8 hours	Servings: 8

Ingredients

- Beef chuck roast – 1 ½ lb.
- Sliced fresh button or cremini mushrooms – 3 cups
- Chopped onion – 1 cup
- Garlic – 4 cloves, minced
- Salt – ½ tsp.
- Black pepper – ½ tsp.
- Quick-cooking tapioca -1/4 cup, crushed
- 50% less-sodium beef broth – 2 (14.5 oz.) cans
- Dry sherry – ½ cup
- Sugar snap pea pods – 4 cups
- Cherry tomatoes – 2 cups, halved
- Hot cooked multigrain noodles – 4 cups

Method

1. Cut meat into ¾-inch pieces.
2. Coat a skillet with cooking spray. Cook meat, half at a time, in the hot skillet until browned.

3. Combine the next five ingredients (through pepper) in a slow cooker. Sprinkle with tapioca. Add meat and pour in broth and dry sherry.
4. Cover and cook on low for 8 to 10 hours or high for 4 to 5 hours.
5. If slow cooker is on low, turn to high. Stir in sugar snap peas. Cover and cook for 5 minutes.
6. Stir in cherry tomatoes. Serve meat mixture over hot cooked noodles.

Nutritional Facts Per Serving

o   Calories: 208

o   Fat: 4g

o   Carb: 19g

o   Protein: 24g

Prep time: 10 minutes	Cook time: 15 minutes	Servings: 4

Ingredients

- Lemon – 1

- Boneless beef shoulder top blade steaks (flat iron) – 2 (6 to 8 oz.)

- Salt – ¼ tsp.

- Black pepper – ¼ tsp.

- Dried rosemary – 1 tsp. crushed

- Olive oil – 4 tsp.

- Grape tomatoes – 2 cups, halved

- Garlic – 2 cloves, minced

- Pitted green olives – 1/3 cup, halved

- Crumbled feta cheese – ¼ cup

- Lemon wedges

Method

1. Remove 1 tsp. zest from the lemon. Set zest aside. Cut steaks in half and season with salt and pepper. Sprinkle rosemary on both sides of the steaks.

2. Heat 2 tsps. oil in a skillet. Add steaks and cook until medium rare, about 8 to 10 minutes. Turning once. Remove and set aside.

3. Add remaining 2 tsps. oil to the skillet. Add garlic and tomatoes. Cook until tomatoes are soft and burst, for about 3 minutes. Remove from heat. Stir in the lemon zest and olives.

4. Serve steaks with tomato relish.

5. Sprinkle with cheese and serve with the reserved lemon wedges.

Nutritional Facts Per Serving

- o   Calories: 223

- o   Fat: 14g

- o   Carb: 6g

- o   Protein: 20g

Spiced Burgers with Cilantro Cucumber Sauce

Prep time: 25 minutes	Cook time: 15 minutes	Servings: 4

Ingredients

- o Plain fat-free Greek yogurt – 1 (5.3 to 6 oz.) container
- o Finely chopped cucumber – 2/3 cup
- o Snipped fresh cilantro – ¼ cup
- o Garlic – 2 cloves, minced
- o Salt – 1/8 tsp.
- o Black pepper – 1/8 tsp.
- o Canned garbanzo beans – ½ cup, rinsed and drained
- o Lean ground beef – 1 lb.
- o Finely chopped red onion – ¼ cup
- o Chopped jalapeno pepper – 2 Tbsps.
- o Salt – ½ tsp.
- o Ground cumin – ¼ tsp.
- o Ground coriander – ¼ tsp.
- o Cinnamon – 1/8 tsp.
- o Black pepper – 1/8 tsp.
- o Radicchio – 1 head, shredded

Method

1. To make the sauce: in a bowl, stir together the first six ingredients (through black pepper). Cover and keep in the refrigerator.
2. In a bowl, mash garbanzo beans with a fork. Add the next eight ingredients (through black pepper), mix well. Form meat mixture into four ¾ inch thick patties.
3. Grill burgers, covered, over medium 14 to 18 minutes or until done (160F). Turning once.
4. Toss radicchio with additional fresh cilantro leaves.
5. Serve burgers on radicchio, top with sauce.

Nutritional Facts Per Serving

o   Calories: 258

o   Fat: 12g

o   Carb: 8g

o   Protein: 29g

Fish and Seafood Recipes

Caribbean Fish with Mango-Orange Relish

Prep time: 25 minutes	Cook time: 15 minutes	Servings: 6

Ingredients

- o Fresh or frozen skinless barramundi, sea bass, or other whitefish fillets – 2 ½ lb.

- o Navel oranges – 3

- o Large mango – 1, chopped

- o Chopped roasted red sweet pepper – ¾ cup

- o Dry white wine – 2 Tbsps.

- o Snipped fresh cilantro – 1 Tbsp.

- o Salt – ¼ tsp.

- o Black pepper – ¼ tsp.

- o All-purpose flour – 1/3 cup

- o Ground cardamom – 2 tsps.

- o Butter – ¼ cup

- o Snipped fresh chives

Method

1. For relish, juice one of the oranges. Peel and section the remaining two oranges. Combine orange sections, orange juice and the next four ingredients (through cilantro).
2. Sprinkle fish with salt and pepper. In a dish, combine cardamom and flour. Dip fish in flour mixture, turning to coat.
3. Preheat oven to 300F. In a skillet, melt 2 tbsps. butter. Add half of the fish. Cook until fish is golden and flakes easily, about 6 to 8 minutes. Turning once.
4. Cook the remaining fish in remaining 2 Tbsps. butter. Serve with relish and sprinkle with chives.

Nutritional Facts Per Serving

o   Calories: 343

o   Fat: 12g

o   Carb: 20g

o   Protein: 37g

Lemon-Herb Roasted Salmon Sheet-Pan Dinner

Prep time: 20 minutes	Cook time: 15 minutes	Servings: 4

Ingredients

- o   Fresh or frozen skinless salmon fillet – 1 (1 lb.)
- o   Olive oil – 2 Tbsps.
- o   Dried oregano – 1 ½ tsp. crushed
- o   Salt – ¼ tsp.
- o   Black pepper – 1/8 tsp.
- o   Grape or cherry tomatoes – 2 cups halved
- o   Broccoli florets – 2 cups
- o   Garlic – 2 cloves, minced
- o   Lemon – 1
- o   Snipped fresh basil – 2 Tbsp.
- o   Snipped fresh parsley – 1 Tbsp.
- o   Honey – 1 Tbsp.

Method

1. Thaw salmon, if frozen. Preheat oven to 400F.
2. Line a baking pan with parchment paper.
3. Rinse fish and pat dry.
4. Place salmon in the prepared pan. Drizzle with 1 tbsp. oil and sprinkle with ¾ tsp. oregano, salt and pepper.

5. In a bowl, combine garlic, broccoli, tomatoes, and remaining 1 tbsp. oil and ¾ tsp. oregano. Sprinkle lightly with more salt and pepper. Toss to coat.
6. Place in the pan with salmon. Roast until salmon flakes, about 15 to 18 minutes.
7. Meanwhile, remove 1 tsp. zest and squeeze 3 tbsps. juice from lemon. In a small bowl, combine lemon juice and zest and remaining ingredients.
8. Spoon over salmon and vegetables before serving.

Nutritional Facts Per Serving

o Calories: 276

o Fat: 14g

o Carb: 13g

o Protein: 25g

Prep time: 10 minutes	Cook time: 5 minutes	Servings: 6

Ingredients

- Frozen peeled, cooked shrimp – 1 (6 oz.) pkg. thawed and finely chopped
- Chopped cooked chicken – ½ cup
- Chopped fresh mushrooms – ½ cup
- Reduced-sodium soy sauce – 2 Tbsps.
- Sliced green onions – ½ cup
- Snipped fresh cilantro – ¼ cup
- Wonton wrappers – 24
- Low-sodium chicken broth – 6 cups
- Chopped red sweet pepper – ¾ cup
- Frozen edamame – ½ cup
- Salt – ¼ tsp.
- Fresh baby spinach – 2 cups
- Toasted sesame oil – 2 tsps.

Method

1. For filling, combine the first four ingredients (through soy sauce), ¼ cup of the green onions, and 2 tsps. cilantro.
2. Working with two wonton wrappers at a time, top each with a rounded tsp. of the filling. Brush edges of the wrappers with water. Fold and seal edges. Repeat with the remaining.
3. In a saucepan, combine the next four ingredients (through salt) and the remaining green onions and cilantro.
4. Bring to a boil. Slowly add wontons to boiling broth mixture. Boil gently until tender, about 2 to 3 minutes. Stirring occasionally.
5. Stir in sesame oil and spinach.
6. Top with additional snipped fresh cilantro and serve.

Nutritional Facts Per Serving

o Calories: 189

o Fat: 3g

o Carb: 24g

o Protein: 17g

Cod with Eggplant Peperonata

Prep time: 10 minutes	Cook time: 25 minutes	Servings: 4

Ingredients

- Fresh or frozen cod fillets – 4 (4-oz.)
- Medium sweet onion – ½, thinly sliced
- Olive oil – 1 Tbsp.
- Small eggplant – 1, cut into 1-inch pieces
- Yellow or red sweet pepper – 1 large, thinly sliced
- Garlic – 4 cloves, minced
- Snipped fresh rosemary – 1 tsp.
- Salt – ½ tsp.
- Black pepper – ¼ tsp.
- Fresh spinach – 4 cups

Method

1. Thaw fish, if frozen. Rinse fish, pat dry with paper towels.
2. For eggplant peperonata, in a skillet, cook onion in hot oil for 5 minutes. Stirring occasionally.
3. Add the next four ingredients (through rosemary), and ¼ tsp. salt. Cook until vegetables are very tender, about 10 to 12 minutes. Stirring occasionally. Remove peperonata from skillet and keep warm.

4. Add 1-inch of water to the same skillet. Place a steamer basket in the skillet and bring the water to boil. Sprinkle cod with the remaining ¼ tsp. salt and the black pepper.
5. Add fish to the steamer basket. Cover and reduce heat to medium. Steam just until fish flakes, about 6 to 8 minutes.
6. Top spinach with fish and eggplant peperonata.

Nutritional Facts Per Serving

o Calories: 189

o Fat: 5g

o Carb: 13g

o Protein: 23g

Prep time: 20 minutes	Cook time: 20 minutes	Servings: 4

Ingredients

- Fresh or frozen skinless cod fillets – 4 (5 to 6 oz.) fillets

- Small zucchini or yellow summer squash – 4, cut into ¾ inch pieces

- Garlic – 2 cloves, minced

- Olive oil – ¼ cup

- Salt – ¼ tsp.

- Black pepper – 1/8 tsp.

- Panko breadcrumbs – ¼ cup

- Grated Parmesan cheese – ¼ cup

- Snipped fresh parsley – 2 Tbsp.

Method

1. Preheat the oven to 350F. in a baking pan, combine garlic and squash.
2. Drizzle with 2 tbsp. oil. Rinse and pat dry fish. Place in pan with squash. Sprinkle fish and squash with 1/8 tsp. of the salt and pepper.

3. In a bowl, combine parsley, cheese, panko, and remaining 1/8 tsp. salt. Drizzle with the remaining 2 tbsp. oil and toss to coat.
4. Sprinkle eon top of the fish. Press lightly.
5. Bake for about 20 minutes or until fish flakes.
6. Sprinkle with additional parsley.
7. Serve.

Nutritional Facts Per Serving

- Calories: 297

- Fat: 16g

- Carb: 8g

- Protein: 29g

Fried Cauliflower Rice with Shrimp

Prep time: 10 minutes	Cook time: 10 minutes	Servings: 4

Ingredients

- Fresh or frozen medium shrimp – 8 oz. peeled and deveined

- Cauliflower – 1 (2 lb.) head, cut into florets

- Toasted sesame oil – 1 tsp.

- Eggs – 2, lightly beaten

- Olive oil – 1 Tbsp.

- Grated fresh ginger – 4 tsp.

- Garlic – 4 cloves, minced

- Chopped napa cabbage – 2 cups

- Coarsely shredded carrots – 1 cup

- Sea salt – ½ tsp.

- Crushed red pepper – ½ tsp.

- Sliced green onions – 1/3 cup

- Snipped fresh cilantro – 2 Tbsp.

- Lime wedges

Method

1. Thaw shrimp if frozen. Rinse shrimp and pat dry.
2. Pulse cauliflower in a food processor until rice size.
3. In a skillet, heat sesame oil over medium heat. Add eggs, stir gently until set. Remove eggs and cool slightly. Cut eggs into strips.
4. Heat the olive oil in the skillet over medium heat. Add garlic and ginger. Cook for 30 seconds.
5. Add carrots and cabbage and stir-fry until vegetables start to soften, about 2 minutes.
6. Add crushed red pepper, salt, and shrimp. Stir-fry for 2 minutes or until shrimp are opaque.
7. Add green onions, and cooked egg. Stir-fry until heated through.
8. Shrink shrimp mixture with cilantro. Serve with lemon wedges.

Nutritional Facts Per Serving

- Calories: 181

- Fat: 8g

- Carb: 14g

- Protein: 17g

Quick Scallop and Noodle Toss

Prep time: 5 minutes	Cook time: 10 minutes	Servings: 4

Ingredients

- o Fresh or frozen sea scallops – 12
- o Medium zucchini – 1, trimmed
- o Olive oil – ½ tsp.
- o Orange juice – 2 Tbsps.
- o Cider vinegar – 2 Tbsps.
- o Toasted sesame oil – 1 Tbsp.
- o Grated fresh ginger – 1 tsp.
- o Lime zest – ½ tsp.
- o Sea salt – ½ tsp.
- o Fresh baby spinach – 1 ½ cups
- o Chopped cucumber – 1 cup
- o Thinly sliced radishes – 2/3 cups
- o Black pepper – ¼ tsp.
- o Olive oil – 1 Tbsp.
- o Sesame seeds – 2 Tbsps. toasted

Method

1. Thaw scallops, if frozen. Cut zucchini into long, thin noodles.
2. Heat ½ tsp. olive oil in a skillet. Add zucchini noodles and stir-fry for 1 minute or until tender. Cool.
3. Meanwhile, in a bowl, combine the next five ingredients (through lime zest) and ¼ tsp. salt. Stir in radishes, cucumber, spinach, and zucchini noodles.
4. Rinse scallops and pat dry. Sprinkle with remaining ¼ tsp. salt and pepper.
5. Heat 1 tbsp. olive oil in the same skillet. Add the scallops and cook until opaque, about 3 to 5 minutes. Turning once.
6. Serve zucchini noodle mixture with scallops and sprinkle with sesame seeds.

Nutritional Facts Per Serving

o   Calories: 227

o   Fat: 10g

o   Carb: 9g

o   Protein: 24g

Meatless/Vegan Recipes

Falafel and Vegetable Pitas

Prep time: 25 minutes	Cook time: 5 minutes	Servings: 4

Ingredients

- Lemon – 1
- Reduced-sodium garbanzo beans – 1 (15-oz.)can, rinsed and drained
- Whole-wheat flour – 2 Tbsps.
- Snipped fresh Italian parsley – 2 Tbsps.
- Garlic – 3 cloves, sliced
- Ground coriander – ½ tsp.
- Salt – ¼ tsp.
- Black pepper – ¼ tsp.
- Ground cumin – 1/8 tsp.
- Whole grain pita bread rounds – 2, halved
- Fresh spinach or watercress – ¾ cup
- Roma tomato – 8 thin slices
- Thinly sliced cucumber – ½ cup
- Yogurt sauce – 1 recipe

Method

1. Remove 2 tsps. zest and squeeze 2 tbsps. juice from lemon.
2. To make the falafel, in a food processor, combine the juice, zest, and the next eight ingredients (through cumin). Cover and process until finely chopped.
3. Shape garbanzo bean mixture into four ½-inch thick oval patties. Coat a skillet with cooking spray and heat over medium heat.
4. Add patties and cook until browned, for about 4 to 6 minutes. Turning once.
5. Open pita halves to make pockets. Fill pockets with cucumber slices, tomato slices, and spinach.
6. Add falafel and top with yogurt sauce.
7. Serve.

To make the yogurt sauce: in a bowl stir together ½ cup plain fat-free yogurt, 1/8 tsp. each of salt, and black pepper, and 2 tbsp. fresh Italian parsley.

Nutritional Facts Per Serving

o   Calories: 217

o   Fat: 3g

o   Carb: 43g

o   Protein: 11g

Prep time: 10 minutes	Cook time: 25 minutes	Servings: 6

Ingredients

- o   Unsalted raw cashews – 1/3 cup

- o   Boiling water

- o   Dried whole grain or brown rice fettuccine – 12 oz.

- o   Chopped fresh asparagus – 1 cup

- o   Lightly packed fresh spinach or arugula – 2 cups

- o   Frozen peas – ½ cup, slightly thawed

- o   Water – 1 ¼ cup

- o   Garbanzo bean – ¼ cup, flour

- o   Lemon juice – 1 Tbsp.

- o   Olive oil – 2 tsps.

- o   Garlic – 2 cloves, minced

- o   Kosher salt and black pepper to taste

- o   Snipped fresh basil – 2 Tbsps.

- o   Shaved parmesan cheese

Method

1. In a small bowl, combine cashews and enough boiling water to cover. Let stand, covered, 20 minutes, then drain. Rinse and drain again.
2. Meanwhile, cook pasta according to package directions. Add asparagus in the last 3 minutes and add spinach and peas in the last 1 minute of cooking. Drain.
3. In a small saucepan, whisk together the flour and water until smooth. Cook and stir over medium heat until just until bubbly.
4. For sauce, in a blender, combine soaked cashews, flour mixture, and the next five ingredients (through pepper). Cover and pulse several times. Then blend until smooth. Transfer pasta mixture to a serving dish.
5. Drizzle with sauce. Toss to coat.
6. Sprinkle with more pepper and parmesan cheese.
7. Serve.

Nutritional Facts Per Serving

- Calories: 290

- Fat: 7g

- Carb: 49g

- Protein: 11g

Mediterranean Fried Quinoa

Prep time: 10 minutes	Cook time: 25 minutes	Servings: 4

Ingredients

- Reduced-sodium chicken broth – 2 cups
- Red quinoa – 1 cup
- Olive oil – 1 Tbsp.
- Eggplant – 3 cups, ½ inch pieces
- Coarsely chopped onion – ¾ cup
- Garlic – 2 cloves, minced
- Black pepper – ¼ tsp.
- Grape tomatoes – 1 cup
- Fresh baby spinach – 4 cups
- Pitted Kalamata olives – ¼ cup, halved
- Snipped fresh oregano – 1 Tbsp.
- Crumbled feta cheese – ¼ cup
- Lemon wedges

Method

1. In a saucepan, bring broth to boiling. Add quinoa and return to boiling. Lower heat, simmer, covered, until liquid is absorbed, about 15 minutes. Remove from

heat. Drain and return quinoa to saucepan. Cook and stir over low heat to dry excess moisture from quinoa.

2. Heat oil in a skillet. Add quinoa and cook until starts to brown, about 2 to 4 minutes. Add pepper, garlic, onion, and eggplant. Stir-fry for 3 minutes.

3. Add tomatoes, and stir-fry for 2 minutes or until tomatoes start to burst. Remove from heat. Add spinach, oregano, and olives. Toss.

4. Sprinkle with feta cheese and serve with lemon wedges.

Nutritional Facts Per Serving

o   Calories: 291

o   Fat: 10g

o   Carb: 41g

o   Protein: 11g

Asparagus and Greens with Farro

Prep time: 10 minutes	Cook time: 30 minutes	Servings: 4

Ingredients

- o Water – 3 cups

- o Uncooked farro – 1 cup

- o Thin asparagus – 1 bunch, trimmed and cut into 2-inch pieces

- o Lemon juice – 3 Tbsps.

- o Whole almonds – ½ cup, toasted and chopped

- o Olive oil – 1 Tbsp.

- o Kosher salt – ½ tsp.

- o Black pepper – ¼ tsp.

- o Baby spinach and/or baby kale – 3 cups

- o Shaved Parmesan cheese – 1/3 cup

Method

1. In a saucepan, bring water to boil. Add farro, lower heat, simmer, covered, until just tender, about 30 minutes. Drain.
2. Meanwhile, place a steamer basket in a skillet. Add water to just below basket. Bring water to boil.
3. Add asparagus to basket. Cover, and steam until crisp-tender, about 3 minutes. Transfer to a large bowl.

4. Add farro to bowl with asparagus. Drizzle with lemon juice and stir in pepper, salt, olive oil, and almonds. Add greens and toss to combine. Top with Parmesan.

Nutritional Facts Per Serving

o   Calories: 360

o   Fat: 15g

o   Carb: 43g

o   Protein: 15g

Toasted Walnut Tempeh Tacos

Prep time: 5 minutes	Cook time: 15 minutes	Servings: 4

Ingredients

o Fresh poblano pepper – 1 medium, seeded and chopped

o Chopped onion – ½ cup

o Tempeh – 1 (8-oz.) pkg. crumbled

o Garlic – 2 cloves, minced

o Salt-free Mexican-seasoning blend – 2 tsps.

o Salt – ¼ tsp.

o Chopped walnuts – ¼ cup, toasted

o Chopped avocado – ½ cup

o Lime juice – ½ tsp.

o Salt – 1/8 tsp.

o Corn tortillas – 8 (6-inch), warmed

o Shredded romaine lettuce – 1 ½ cups

o Refrigerated fresh salsa – 1 cup

o Crumbled Cotija cheese – ¼ cup

o Chopped fresh cilantro – ½ cup

Method

1. Coat a skillet with cooking spray and heat over medium heat.
2. Add onion and pepper and cook until vegetables are crisp-tender, about 3 to 5 minutes. Stirring occasionally.
3. Add the next four ingredients (though salt). Cook until heated and tempeh is lightly browned, about 6 to 8 minutes. Stirring occasionally. Remove from heat and stir in walnuts.
4. Meanwhile, in a small bowl, mash avocado with 1/8 tsp. salt, and lime juice. Spread mashed avocado over tortillas, then top with lettuce.
5. Spoon warm tempeh mixture over lettuce. Top with cilantro, cheese, and salsa.

Nutritional Facts Per Serving

o   Calories: 380

o   Fat: 19g

o   Carb: 37g

o   Protein: 18g

Prep time: 10 minutes	Cook time: 50 minutes	Servings: 6

Ingredients

- Vegetable broth – 2 cups
- Dried brown lentils – ½ cup, rinsed and drained
- Dried rosemary – ½ tsp. crushed
- Dried thyme – ½ tsp. crushed
- Round red potatoes – 2 ½ lb. cut into 1-inch pieces
- Garlic – 2 cloves, peeled
- Butter – 5 Tbsps.
- Salt – ¾ tsp.
- Sliced fresh mushrooms – 3 cups
- Chopped onion – 1 cup
- Frozen peas and carrots – 1 ½ cups
- Reduced-sodium soy sauce – 4 tsps.
- Cornstarch - 1 Tbsp.
- Worcestershire sauce – 2 tsps.

Method

1. Bring 1 cup water to boil in a saucepan. Add lentils, rosemary, and thyme. Simmer, covered, until tender, about 30 to 40 minutes. Drain.
2. Meanwhile, preheat oven to 375F.
3. In a Dutch oven, cook potatoes, and garlic in boiling water until potatoes are tender, about 15 minutes. Drain, and reserve ½ cup cooking water. Coarsely mash potatoes. Mash in the salt and 3 tbsps. butter. Stir in enough reserved cooking water to reach desired consistency.
4. Heat 1 tbsp. butter in a skillet. Add onion and mushrooms and cook for 10 minutes. Stirring occasionally. Stir in carrots and peas.
5. In a small bowl, combine the 1 cup broth, Worcestershire sauce, soy sauce, and cornstarch. Stir into the mushroom mixture.
6. Stir-fry until thickened and bubbly. Cook and stir 1 minute more. Stir in cooked lentils.
7. Top lentil mixture with mashed potatoes, spreading to edges. Dot with remaining 1 tbsp. butter.
8. Transfer skillet to the oven and bake until potatoes start to brown, about 20 minutes.

Nutritional Facts Per Serving

o   Calories: 328

o   Fat: 10g

o   Carb: 51g

o   Protein: 11g

Prep time: 15 minutes	Cook time: 30 minutes	Servings: 1

Ingredients

- o Reduced-sodium chicken broth – 1 cup
- o Steel-cut oats – ½ cup
- o Toasted sesame oil – 2 tsps.
- o Assorted fresh mushrooms – 1 cup, sliced
- o Minced fresh ginger – 1 tsp.
- o Green onions – 2, cut into 1-inch pieces
- o Reduced-sodium soy sauce – 1 tsp.
- o Crushed red pepper

Method

1. Bring broth to a boil in a saucepan. Stir in oats. Reduce heat to medium-low. Cook, uncovered, until oats are tender, and mixture is thickened and creamy, about 25 to 30 minutes. Stirring occasionally.
2. Meanwhile, heat 1 tsp. oil in a skillet. Add ginger and mushrooms and cook until tender, about 3 to 4 minutes. Transfer to a bowl.
3. Add remaining oil to skillet. Increase heat to medium-high. Add green onions and cook until charred, about 2 minutes. Remove from heat.
4. Stir mushrooms into oats.

5. Top with crushed red pepper, green onions, and soy sauce.
6. Serve.

Nutritional Facts Per Serving

o   Calories: 474

o   Fat: 15g

o   Carb: 65g

o   Protein: 21g

Desserts

Frozen Yogurt Bark

Prep time: 15 minutes	Freeze time: 2 hours	Servings: 24

Ingredients

- o   Plain Whole-milk Greek yogurt – 1 (32-oz.) carton
- o   Honey – ¼ cup
- o   Vanilla extract – 2 tsp.
- o   Filling – 1 cup (chopped berries, nuts, dark chocolate)
- o   Toppers – 2 cups (cacao nibs, seeds, nuts, fruit, toasted raw chip coconut)

Method

1. Line two large baking sheet with parchment paper. In a bowl, combine vanilla, honey, and yogurt. Stir in fillings.
2. Divide yogurt mixture between prepared baking sheets, spreading into rectangles. Sprinkle with toppers.
3. Freeze 2 to 4 hours or until firm. Break bark into 24 irregular pieces.
4. Serve.

Nutritional Facts Per Serving

- o   Calories: 117

- o Fat: 7g
- o Carb: 9g
- o Protein: 5g

Sweet Ricotta and Strawberry Parfaits

Prep time: 10 minutes	Cook time: 0 minutes	Servings: 6

Ingredients

- Fresh strawberries – 1 lb. quartered
- Snipped fresh mint – 1 Tbsp.
- Sugar – 1 tsp.
- Part-skim ricotta cheese – 1 (15-oz.) carton
- Honey – 3 Tbsps.
- Vanilla – ½ tsp.
- Lemon zest – ¼ tsp.

Method

1. In a bowl, stir together sugar, mint, and strawberries. Let stand until berries are softened, about 15 minutes.
2. In a bowl, beat the remaining ingredients with a mixer for 2 minutes.
3. To assemble: scoop about 2 tbsps. ricotta mixture into each parfait glass. Top each with a large spoonful of strawberry mixture. Repeat layers.
4. Top with additional fresh mint. Serve.

Nutritional Facts Per Serving

- Calories: 159
- Fat: 6g

- Carb: 18g
- Protein: 9g

Chocolate-Date Truffles

Prep time: 10 minutes	Freeze time: 1 hour	Servings: 10

Ingredients

- Coarsely chopped walnuts – ½ cup
- Salt – 1/8 tsp.
- Pitted whole Medjool dates – 1 ½ cups
- Unsweetened cocoa powder – 3 Tbsps.
- Apple juice – 1 Tbsp.
- Salt – ¼ tsp.
- Water
- Cocoa powder

Method

1. Process walnuts and 1/8 tsp. salt in a food processor until finely chopped. Transfer to a bowl.
2. Combine the next four ingredients (through ¼ tsp. salt) in the food processor. Pulse until mixture forms a thick paste. Add water if necessary.
3. For each truffle, shape 2 tsp. of the mixture into a ball. Roll balls in walnuts to coat. Chill for 15 to 20 minutes. Dust with cocoa powder.
4. Cover and chill 1 hour and serve.

Nutritional Facts Per Serving

- Calories: 105

- Fat: 4g

- Carb: 19g

- Protein: 2g

Prep time: 10 minutes	Cook time: 5 minutes	Servings: 4

Ingredients

- Sugar – ¼ cup
- Cornstarch – 2 Tbsp.
- Low fat (1%) milk – 2 ½ cups
- Egg yolks – 4, lightly beaten
- Orange zest – ½ tsp.
- Vanilla – ½ tsp.
- Coarsely crushed shortbread cookies – ¼ cup
- Orange slices

Method

1. Stir together cornstarch and sugar in a saucepan, stir in milk. Cook until thick and bubbly. Cook and stir 2 minutes more. Remove from heat.
2. Bit-by-bit, stir in about 1 cup of the hot mixture into the egg yolks. Return to saucepan. Bring just to boil and remove from heat.
3. Stir in orange zest and vanilla. Pour into a serving bowl or four dessert dishes and cover surface with plastic wrap. Cool slightly.
4. Chill at least 4 hours before serving. Do not stir.
5. Top custard with crushed cookies and orange slices.

6. Serve.

Nutritional Facts Per Serving

o   Calories: 212

o   Fat: 7g

o   Carb: 28g

o   Protein: 8g

Creamy Chocolate Pudding

Prep time: 5 minutes	Cook time: 0 minutes	Servings: 4

Ingredients

- o Ripe avocado – 1, peeled and cut up
- o Banana – ½, peeled and cut up
- o Unsweetened cocoa powder – ½ cup
- o Milk – ½ cup
- o Honey – 3 to 4 Tbsps.
- o Vanilla – 2 tsps.

Method

1. Combine all the ingredients in a blender. Blend until smooth. Chill and serve.

Nutritional Facts Per Serving

- o Calories: 163
- o Fat: 7g
- o Carb: 26g
- o Protein: 4g

Prep time: 10 minutes	Cook time: 5 minutes	Servings: 45

Ingredients

- Semisweet chocolate pieces – 1 ¼ cups
- Butterscotch-flavor pieces – ½ cup
- Fat-free half-and-half – 1/3 cup
- Unsalted peanuts – 1 cup
- Baked miniature frozen phyllo shells -45
- Unsalted peanuts – ¼ cup, finely chopped
- Flaked sea salt

Method

1. Melt the butterscotch-flavor pieces, and chocolate pieces in a saucepan. Stirring frequently and melt until smooth. Stir in half-and-half until smooth. Stir in the 1 cup peanuts.
2. Quickly spoon peanut mixture into phyllo shells (using about 2 tsp. per shell).
3. Before mixture is set, sprinkle tops with the finely chopped peanuts and flakes sea salt.
4. Let stand at room temperature for 15 minutes and serve.

Nutritional Facts Per Serving

- o Calories: 85
- o Fat: 5g
- o Carb: 8g
- o Protein: 2g

Apricot Pocket Cookies

Prep time: 1 hour	Cook time: 10 minutes	Servings: 24

Ingredients

- Butter – 1/3 cup, softened
- Granulated sugar – ½ cup
- Baking powder – ¾ tsp.
- Salt – ¼ tsp.
- Light sour cream - ¼ cup
- Egg – 1
- Vanilla – 1 tsp.
- Cake four – 2 2/3 cups, sifted
- Dried apricots – ¾ cup
- Granulated sugar – 1 ½ Tbsps.
- Powdered sugar – 1 cup
- Fat-free milk – 3 to 4 tsps.
- Almond extract – 1 tsp.

Method

1. Beat butter with a mixture in a bowl for 30 seconds. Add ½ cup sugar, salt, and baking powder. Beat until combined. Add vanilla, egg, and sour cream. Beat

154

until combined. Beat in flour. Divide dough in half. Cover and chill dough about 1 ½ hours.

2. In another bowl, combine apricots and enough boiling water to cover. Let stand for 1 hour. Drain and pat dry apricots. Finely chop. Combine apricots and 1 ½ tbsps. sugar.

3. Preheat oven to 375F.

4. Lightly flour your work surface. Roll half of the dough to 1/8 inch thick. Cut dough into rounds with a cookie cutter.

5. Arrange half the cutouts 1 inch apart on ungreased cookie sheets. Brush outer edges of cutout with water. Spoon rounded teaspoons of apricot mixture in centers of cutouts on cookie sheets. Lay remaining cutouts over filling. Lightly press edges of assembled cooking to seal.

6. Bake until firm and bottoms are lightly browned, about 8 to 9 minutes. Remove and cool on wire racks. Repeat with the remaining dough and filling.

7. For icing, in a bowl, stir together the remaining ingredients; add more milk, 1 tsp. at a time, to reach drizzling consistency.

8. Drizzle icing on cooled cookies.

Nutritional Facts Per Serving

o   Calories: 132

o   Fat: 3g

o   Carb: 25g

o   Protein: 2g

Conclusion

Diabetes can be an annoying condition with lots of limitations and risks, however, it doesn't have to be a life sentence. Awareness is the first step to making conscious change. The next step is to be determined to make a conscious change. Develop a plan and jump into action. There are several things that you can do in order to control diabetes, the most important and perhaps the most powerful one of them is modifying your dietary habits. We hope that you have found our guidance on low carb foods, foods to seek and foods to avoid helpful in your journey to combat diabetes.

Printed in Great Britain
by Amazon